NATIONAL HEALTH CRISIS

NATIONAL HEALTH CRISIS
CRISIS
A MODERN SOLUTION

RAY WHITNEY
O.B.E., M.P.

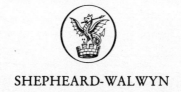

SHEPHEARD-WALWYN

ISBN 0 85683 099 2

Printed and bound in Great Britain
for Shepheard-Walwyn (Publishers) Ltd,
26 Charing Cross Road (Suite 34), London WC2H 0DH
by Cox & Wyman Ltd, Reading, Berkshire,
from typesetting by Alacrity Phototypesetters,
Banwell Castle, Weston-super-Mare.

Cover design by Alan Downs
Photo from Image Bank

To my wife,
Sheila

Contents

	Preface	1
1	Safe in Whose Hands?	5
2	Making the Myth	16
3	Bevan's Bill	34
4	'Cascades of Medicine'	45
5	Changing the Structure	65
6	Can We Make the Straitjacket More Comfortable?	81
7	How Much Does the Health Service 'Need'?	96
8	What Can We Learn from Others?	109
9	Some Roads Worth Exploring	127
10	A Modern Solution to an Old Problem	138
	References	159
	Index	163

Preface

When I began this book in the summer of 1987 my hope was that it might help to start a national debate on how we could provide a modern and comprehensive health service which would best meet the needs of a prosperous but caring society. Having spent two years as a Minister in the Department of Health and Social Security, I had become convinced that the National Health Service, created in 1948 in a very different society, could not measure up to that challenge.

During the election campaign in May and June of 1987 and in the months that followed, Margaret Thatcher and the Conservative Government stuck to the theme that "the NHS is safe in our hands — and only in our hands". As concern about the health service mounted, that cry became more desperate — and still less convincing.

Labour and the other political parties did what all British politicians out of office have been doing for forty years — fiercely attacked the Government for their desecration of a national monument, the NHS. Many working inside the health service provided them with an endless supply of ammunition.

The battle raged and the media loved it. The Government found still more money for the NHS but morale in the service continued to plummet. Everyone shouted the same old things from the same old positions.

Then, quite suddenly, the situation began to change. More people came to accept the Government's claim that, thanks to a

1

healthy economy, they were spending much more than ever before on the NHS. The Government found itself forced to face the possibility that, without a major reform, the health service would be safe in no-one's hands — not even those of the Conservative Party. The shouting continued unabated but the thinking had started.

It is my ambition that this book will contribute to that process. It is written from the position of one who arrived at the DHSS believing that the NHS could be made to work better but that it was the system that was right for Britain — the position of every Health Minister, Labour and Conservative, since 1948. It springs from the frustration I witnessed and experienced during my time at the Department: the frustration of many thousands of people working within the NHS and totally committed to its ideals who know how much better would be the service they provide if only they had the resources; and the frustration of Ministers who dedicate more and more public funds to the NHS and try to ensure that they are used more effectively, only to meet with contumely and despair.

One of the problems has been that there has been too little knowledge and too little thinking. Knowledge of what went on in the past and what is being achieved in health care in other countries today has largely been kept to a small group of specialists. New thinking about the NHS has been minimal. It has been tabooed by the NHS insiders, both because of their emotional commitment to the concept and because they believe the *status quo* best serves their interests (all of us act from complex motives most of the time). And it has been tabooed by the politicians, primarily because they are well aware of the mystic power that the NHS, despite all its failures, still holds over the British public but also because Ministers, who ought to understand the dilemma, have time only to try to make the system work a little better.

I hope what follows will go at least a small way towards filling those gaps. It is based on a year's reflection and study after being removed from the DHSS and a recognition that we shall only be able to create health services which the British people now have a right to expect if we can examine the problems — and the possibilities — calmly, rationally and free of preconceptions. Worrying as the situation in the NHS may now seem to be, there are other time bombs ticking away beneath it which give *us* very little time. We now have to think — and act — very quickly.

I owe a debt of gratitude to many who have helped me in the preparation of this book. I should first mention all those in the DHSS and the NHS who have given me instruction, advice and friendship. I hope the national debate which is now under way will make their professional lives easier and more rewarding than they are at present. I am particularly grateful to the Library Staff of the House of Commons for the exemplary manner in which they have responded to my flood of requests over many months. My thanks are also due to Dr Kenneth Groom, Dr Michael Goldsmith, Bob Beveridge, Hugh Elwell, John Peet, Michael Powell, James Webber, David Boddy, my publisher Anthony Werner and my secretary Caroline Roberts — and many more.

But let me end this preface with the disclaimer offered, in jest, by Joseph Epstein in one of his essays in *The Middle of My Tether*:

"I wrote this book in the hope of making a persuasive argument, while giving pleasure to myself in forming my thoughts into sentences, paragraphs and chapters. Whether I shall give anything even resembling an equivalent pleasure to my readers is highly doubtful, I realize, but an author retains his slender hopes. I wish my book were better than it is, but I fear that it is quite the best that I have had the skill and patience to make. If any justification of the book is needed, it is that the book seeks, in its stuttering way, to take a very small part in a conversation which has been going on for a very long while now. For myself, I hope to be able to read it ten years hence without shame or regret."

He was joking. I mean it.

RAY WHITNEY
Sunninghill, January 1988

1

Safe in Whose Hands?

In the bright after-glow of the Conservative Party's third successive election victory in June 1987 it became easy to forget that there was a point in the campaign when Margaret Thatcher and her closest advisers suddenly realised that defeat was, after all, a real possibility. The City took the same view and over £6 billion were wiped off share values in an hour.

This trauma occurred on 4th June 1987, a date that has entered British political history as "wobbly Thursday". It happened because that was the day that the Labour Party decided to play the NHS card — which quickly proved to be far more damaging to the Conservatives than unemployment or any of the other issues which had emerged during the campaign. It was yet another demonstration of the potency of the NHS phenomenon which has cast its extraordinary spell over British politics for forty years.

Neil Kinnock began the day with a visit to St Thomas's Hospital, London. This created just the sort of "photo-opportunities" he was after as he stimulated and reinforced the complaints of the staff and patients about the way the hospital had been "underfunded" by an uncaring Tory government.

He then went back over Westminster Bridge to launch one of the few press conferences Labour risked holding in London during the election campaign. Kinnock's advisers had, rightly, decided that for the most part he would find the media easier to handle at meetings in the provinces but today was different. They had discovered a health story which might have been designed for Kinnock's special talent for mawkish sentimentality and was a perfect vehicle to underline Labour's claim to be the only true believer in and defender of the National Health Service. This is a claim which, despite a mass of tangible evidence to the contrary, has been widely accepted since 1948 and has therefore become a *political* fact, as regularly demonstrated in four decades of opinion polls.

Labour's campaign managers had just been told of the problems of Mark Burgess, a ten-year-old Kent boy who had been waiting 15 months for a hole-in-the-heart operation. Mark had been scheduled to be admitted to Guy's Hospital a few days earlier but, almost at the last minute, Guy's had been obliged to postpone his treatment, judging that, whilst his condition was serious, he was not in such urgent need as some of their other patients.

At his press conference Kinnock milked the story for all it was worth, conjuring up all the old myths and demons which have haunted the health service since his fellow Welshman, Aneurin Bevan, created it. Only Labour really understood and genuinely believed in the NHS, whilst the Conservatives, notwithstanding all the resources they had diverted to it over the years, secretly intended that it should wither away.

Margaret Thatcher was tackled on the Burgess case at her own press conference minutes after Kinnock had made his attack and was immediately thrown on the defensive. All she could suggest was that Mark should write to her about his problem. She was then led on to her own use of private health insurance facilities and responded that she did so "to enable me to go into hospital on the day I want, at the time I want and with the doctor I want." The proposition that the head of government should enjoy such a freedom would surely be questioned in no other country in the world, whatever the political system, but in Britain this was dangerous political ground indeed. Although some 5 million Britons have similar insurance benefits, the Prime Minister's phrase was seized on to haunt and damage her throughout the rest of the election campaign and beyond.

The *Daily Mirror*, the most persistent and unscrupulous critic of the Conservatives and their custodianship of the NHS, gleefully took up the Mark Burgess story and Thatcher's suggestion that he write to her. The *Mirror*'s health correspondent, Jill Palmer, was despatched to "help" Mark and his grandmother compose a letter to the Prime Minister. This duly appeared on the paper's front page the following day under the gleeful legend: "You asked for it Prime Minister ... the letter that shames your Government." Miss Palmer had fully earned Mr Maxwell's money for the help she gave Mark with his appeal ... "Please can you help me. I have got a bad heart and am sick. I want to know when they are going to make me better. I want to grow up ... I want to get better. Can you get the doctors to make me better?"

All of us who fought the 1987 election under the Conservative banner knew that health would be our most vulnerable flank. We had therefore prepared our defensive material and it was particularly familiar to me as a former Health Minister. For two years I had used it constantly on the national media and on dozens of official excursions around the country. From the Prime Minister downwards every Conservative candidate pointed again and again to the 31% increase in government spending on health, even after allowing for inflation, in the eight years since we had come to office; cited the 10,000 more doctors and dentists, the 63,000 nurses and midwives, all now paid significantly more for a shorter working week and the millions more patients being treated in our hospitals each year.

Yet even many of those who were prepared to accept our statistics were nevertheless convinced that the NHS was collapsing and that nurses, still grossly underpaid, were leaving in droves. They were disposed to believe that the fundamental cause of these ills was that, despite all our protestations and expenditure of national resources, Conservatives were not genuinely committed to the Health Service.

The Conservative Party therefore lost the battle on health during the 1987 campaign. Fortunately what we had to offer in other areas and the unattractiveness of the Labour Party enabled us to win the election. Tory policies to combat inflation, promote economic growth, curb the powers of the trade unions and spread home and share ownership had all been demonstrably successful. The electorate was not persuaded that the policies of the Opposition parties were likely to reduce unemployment more rapidly or effectively than ours were. Most important of all, a majority of voters believed that national security would be seriously jeopardised if entrusted to the Labour Party.

After its resounding victory, the Conservative Government gave little indication that it really understood the magnitude of the problem and still less that it was prepared to contemplate significant changes in the delivery of health care in this country. The Party had campaigned on a programme which showed that it fully recognised that the task it set itself in 1979 to revitalise Britain was still far from complete and the Queen's Speech after the election duly listed a set of suitably radical and exciting proposals. The new Government pledged itself to more tax cuts, privatisation and trade union reform, to greater competition in the provision of local authority services, to freeing the market in rented housing, to a major shake-up in education and to sweeping changes in the rating system.

A formidable list indeed. Yet its very scope and boldness threw into even sharper relief the *timorousness of this reforming Government's approach to health and social security, which account for very nearly half of all government spending.* The Queen's Speech promised only that her Ministers would "maintain and improve the health and social services."

There could have been no clearer demonstration of the power of the NHS myth which has befogged British politics and the national economy for well over a generation. Here was a massively self-confident Prime Minister, heady with the triumph of her third successive election victory, emboldened with another three-figure majority in the House of Commons and relishing her reputation as a slayer of dragons actually refusing to do battle with by far the most menacing of the dragons that survived. She had tackled many of the nationalised industries, regarded unquestioningly by her

Labour and Conservative predecessors as an inescapable and permanent drain on the national exchequer and had turned them into engines of efficiency, innovation and wealth-creation in the private sector. She had destroyed the dead hand of the consensus which had held that trade union barons, wielding the coercive and supra-legal power of organised labour, must for ever play a major role in a corporate state — and she could, with benefit, have done this even more quickly had she not succumbed to Jim Prior's excessively cautious arguments for a step-by-step approach to trade union reform. And having once been obliged to surrender to Arthur Scargill's miners in 1981, by 1984 she had made the plans and acquired the resolution needed to withstand a miners' strike of unique ferocity, thus demonstrating that an elected government need not be held to ransom by any union — and in the process overturning the long-held political wisdom.

Yet even Mrs Thatcher's courage has regularly deserted her when it has come to facing up to the need to reform the NHS. That instinctive caution which accompanied her boldness and which has enabled her to reach the top of Disraeli's greasy pole has hindered her from confronting the dilemmas surrounding the provision of health care in this country. In the months after the 1987 election her newly-appointed Secretary of State for Social Services, John Moore — a man as likely as any of her Ministers to approach the problems of the NHS with a bold and open mind — made a few tentative intellectual forays into the dangerous arena but she declined either to lead or even to follow him.

A notable example of this was to be found in her speech to the Conservative Party conference in Blackpool in October 1987. It was a rousing performance, judged by *The Times* leader the following day to be "the best she has made to a Conservative conference ... no mean feat". Yet after congratulating the Prime Minister on the way she re-stated her fundamental principles, made clear her determination to improve the quality of education and tackle the problems of the inner cities and on avoiding the temptations of triumphalism, *The Times* was moved to point out that: "She is a remarkable blend of daring and caution. Yesterday she picked her way across the minefield of welfare politics in a gingerly manner. Too gingerly. Mr John Moore deserved a greater lead from the top in his attempt to open up the most important domestic policy debate of present times."

Margaret Thatcher clearly hoped that she would be able to get away with a minimalist approach to the problems of the NHS. Perhaps with a continued effort to improve its housekeeping, a few minor reforms which would be politically painless (or nearly so) and, above all, with the steady increase in health spending which the strengthening economy might permit, a serious look at the issue could be avoided altogether or at least delayed for some years? Surely she and her Ministers could get across to the electorate the excellent Conservative record and the sincerity of her government's commitment to the health service?

Within weeks this assessment was shown to be over-optimistic. The NHS issue exploded with greater violence than ever on the political landscape. The immediate cause, in November 1987, was the case of a Birmingham baby, David Barber. Because of a shortage of intensive care nurses in the West Midlands he was kept waiting for some six weeks for the open heart surgery he needed and when, after much public outrage, the operation finally did take place, he died. The *Daily Mirror* railed against the "cold-hearted" Mrs Thatcher, Labour MPs spoke of "murder" and for many weeks Prime Minister's Question Time in the Commons was massively dominated by the health issue. Neil Kinnock, gratefully seizing on one of the few issues on which his demoralised Party could unite, did everything he could to stoke up the fire. In letters to Mrs Thatcher he warned of 'mounting public anxiety over the condition of the health service", asserted that "the conscience of the nation has rightly been stirred by the many accounts" of postponed operations and complained of the Prime Minister's tendency "to refer to overall figures which fail to answer the specific matters that relate to particular cases."

Margaret Thatcher responded with selections from what had now become her well-known — and increasingly less effective — litany of statistics. "The simple fact is that expenditure on the

NHS has risen from less than £8 billion in 1978-79 to some £21 billion in 1987-88" ... "the cost to the average family ... has increased from £11 a week in 1979 to £29 a week this year". And these additional resources had produced more output ... "out-patient attendances have gone up by over 3 million since 1979 to 38 million last year. The number of heart bypass operations has risen from 265 a month to 880, hip replacements from 2,300 to 3,100 and cataract operations from 3,200 to 4,900."

This line of defence, however, quickly proved to be inadequate. The onslaught continued and public disquiet grew. In what was widely (but incorrectly) believed to be an unprecedented move, the three leaders of the medical profession, the Presidents of the Royal Colleges, issued a strongly-worded call for increased health funding. One consultant who had actually appeared on a Party Political Broadcast for the Conservatives joined the clamour for higher spending. Opinion polls regularly demonstrated that the National Health Service was considered to be the country's most urgent problem and that the level of concern was mounting. BBC Radio 4's "Today" programme reported that the health issue was easily the favourite topic in the letters received from its millions of listeners.

In the face of such pressure the Government felt obliged to yield, if only a little. After the inevitable tussle with the Treasury, the Minister of Health, Tony Newton, was authorised on 16th December 1987 to announce that spending on the hospital and community health services would be increased during the current year (1987-88) by £100 million and that spending in the next financial year would rise by £707 million, a cash increase of 5.7%.

Much more important, however, than yet another increase in NHS resources was the fact that the campaign launched in the Autumn of 1987 by health service insiders, politicians and the media finally began to awaken the nation to the true nature of the problem. It is still very early days — we have been asleep for a long time — but, at last, a readiness to look calmly but critically at the system we have all been trying to make work for forty years was beginning to dawn. Suddenly, new ideas (or at least old or foreign ideas recycled — there is little new in this field) were in the air. The unthinkable could now be thought about, even if the political barriers between the problem and its possible solution still seemed immense and probably insurmountable.

The Prime Minister called for new thinking from the DHSS and her No. 10 Policy Unit — although she remained very cautious about how much change the country would stomach. Her experiences with the health service had left her bruised and baffled (and even, it has been reported, near to tears). From the time her government had taken office in 1979 it had accepted that on a budget it was determined to contain and, if possible, reduce, health service spending was a steadily rising burden, accounting for an ever-higher proportion of our national wealth. For years she had regularly insisted that "the Health Service is safe in our hands" — but this slogan had become a damaging boomerang. In December 1986 I made strong representations that her speech writers should steer her off its use and I believe we were successful for some six months. In the stress of the 1987 election campaign, however, she went back to it. The fact is that the National Health Service as it is currently organised and financed will not much longer be safe in the hands of a government of any persuasion. Reform — and fundamental reform rather than the sort of tinkering that has been tried so far — is essential and urgently needed.

The fallacy at the heart of the National Health Service should have been obvious from its inception — the failure to recognise that the demand for "free" medical care will always quickly outrun any possible provision for it. In the literature and debates of the period it is quite remarkable how little attention was paid to the fundamental issue of resources. Indeed, during the 1940s and even in the 1950s it was a widely-held view across the political parties that as the health of the people became better cared for, spending on the service would actually fall. Of course, the opposite happened and no sooner was it instituted than the NHS began to outstrip all the absurdly optimistic spending projections of its founders. By 1955 public spending on health was accounting for about 3.5% of our gross domestic product and by 1987 it had risen to some 6.2%.

Yet the level of public dissatisfaction with the NHS, and particularly with the delays in hospital treatment, has grown even more vigorously (as opposed to patient satisfaction when they are treated).

The structure of the NHS and the fact that it is funded almost entirely from the national exchequer have always ensured that the provision of health care is a more aggressively politicised issue in Britain than in any other country. For many years we complacently described Bevan's creation as "the envy of the world" — but it is unsurprising that it had no serious imitators.

The NHS arrangements result in Ministers becoming the targets not only of their political opponents but of all those working within the service. The pressure of rising demand on necessarily finite, even though increasing, resources requires that they be rationed and in the health service this rationing is manifested in the length of hospital waiting lists — which then become an effective weapon for Opposition parties to use against Governments. The brouhaha created over Mark Burgess' wait for a "non-urgent" hole-in-the-heart operation and the tragic death of the baby David Barber will be repeated with increasing frequency in the future until real improvements are made in the system.

Those working within the NHS and wishing to squeeze more money out of the Health Minister and the Chancellor of the Exchequer of the day have what Enoch Powell once described as "a vested interest in its denigration". Writing in 1966, following three years as Minister of Health, in a book which carefully delineated the problems but which was surprisingly weak in offering remedies, Powell observed: "Anyone in the National Health Service below the Minister, from the chairman of the hospital board to the nursing anxiliary, who professed himself satisfied with what was being spent could not unreasonably be represented as a traitor to his colleagues, his profession and his patients — on the basis, namely, that more money means improvement and that complaint and dissatisfaction are essential to extracting more money."[1]

The fundamental problems of the NHS which Powell described

a quarter of a century ago and believed then could not "be 'reformed' away while leaving the system as such intact" are now much more acute and will intensify at a geometric rate in the years ahead unless an inescapably painful remedy is quickly prescribed and adopted. Pressure on our health and social services is increasing remorselessly. A major cause is the fact that we are living longer and most of us only start making significant demands on those services once we are into our late sixties and seventies.

As a Health Minister, I visited dozens of hospitals and made a point of asking about the average age in the general — not the geriatric — wards. It usually turned out to be about seventy. A few young men would have broken their legs playing football or falling off their motor-bikes but the majority would nearly always be in their seventies, having their second hip replaced or their cataracts removed. Demography, improving styles of living and more advanced medical care all mean that old age will continue to increase its dominance of the whole health scene.

The pressure on NHS funds is also rising because of the nature of technological advances. The hospital service should now be providing a growing range of equipment which may cost one million pounds an item and operations which, if properly costed (sadly and surprisingly, still an unusual occurrence in the NHS) may be £30,000 each; and these demands will undoubtedly grow. Many doctors, scientists and technicians, naturally and rightly, like to work at the frontiers of their knowledge and skill and constantly extend them. In their fight for the funds they need they will always be able to enlist the passionate support of their patients and families and the general public. The current Aids alarm is adding to these pressures, the cost of preserving the life of a victim even just for a year amounting to around £20,000.

Most of us now aspire to and expect to enjoy good health. Even if we smoke fifty cigarettes a day, drink too much alcohol and never take exercise, we increasingly assume that the Health Service will be able to put us right and believe that, if it does not, politicians have failed to fund or organise it properly. As our perceptions of the powers of modern medicine have been inflated to proportions unjustified at least in the short run, so our readiness to accept the ills to which our flesh is heir has declined.

Given the interest we all have in access to good health care, the huge and growing burden of health spending on the national economy and the political Passchendaele that the issue is now becoming, it is extraordinary that new thinking on the subject has so far been confined very largely to a rather narrow circle of professionals. For the most part there has been a resolute refusal to accept the existence of a problem, let alone a willingness to embark on the search for a solution. Those within the service have clung to the belief (I am sure quite mistakenly) that their interests can best be served by preserving the system and pressing for more resources. Politicians believe, or have affected to believe, that with just a little more money, just a few more reforms and just a little better administration they can postpone grasping the nettle at least for the next few years — for the term, perhaps, of their probable political lives.

So even politicians with the courage of Enoch Powell and Margaret Thatcher have shied away from the challenge of the NHS. As Powell pointed out two decades ago: "Nationalised medical care is virtually insulated from external comparisons by its universality and its free provision to the consumer. The very contemplation of denationalising is enough to daunt the stoutest political heart."[2]

The problems, great as they were then, are now even more daunting but their contemplation — and resolution — can no longer be delayed. Nor, fortified by the prosperity and confidence of the Thatcherite era, should they be. It is now quite clear that the proper management and provision of health care will be one of the crucial issues of British politics in the years ahead — and, indeed, until significant improvements are made.

At last there are signs that a serious search for those improvements is now beginning. That is the process which this book seeks to further.

2
Making the Myth

If we are to find a way to improve the standards of health care in Britain we must start with a realistic appraisal of the strengths and weaknesses of the present system. On any other issue, such a statement would be well into the realms of the banal. In the case of the National Health Service, to aspire to a realistic appraisal will be seen by many as sacrilege and by others (the more charitable) as optimism on a Utopian level.

We are dealing with a unique political and social phenomenon which, whilst bringing many benefits, has also cast a blight on thought and action in this country for forty years. We have taken the reality of the NHS and woven it into a myth; the unravelling of the myth (which need certainly not involve the unravelling of a system of comprehensive health care) will be neither easy nor popular.

It is particularly striking that the myth should have been created here. In Britain we take pride in our down-to-earth level-headedness. Other nations get swept away from time to time by some wave of political hysteria or other. For a decade most Germans seemed to have accepted enthusiastically the doctrines of Hitler and his Nazis. Mussolini had the same effect on the Italians. Hundreds of millions of Russians and Chinese at least *appeared* to have committed themselves wholeheartedly to communism and the worship of Karl Marx, Stalin or Mao Tse-tung. Even in the United States, a large majority were still stubbornly loyal to Ronald

Reagan and his leadership despite all the mistakes and weaknesses revealed during eight years in the White House.

In Britain we have always been much more sceptical, and even cynical, about political ideas and our political leaders. And in recent years that characteristic has grown even stronger. In an increasingly iconoclastic age we can live with or join in attacks on or jokes about all the national institutions our predecessors held dear — the Church, Parliamentary democracy, the freedom of the press, the independence of the judiciary and certainly the nationalised industries and the trade unions. Few, however, have dared to challenge — let alone make jokes about — the fundamental principles of the National Health Service. While it has long been open season on all the other once-sacred cows, the sole survivor has remained very sacred indeed.

The nature of the myth, now forty years in the making, cannot be understood without some knowledge of the facts surrounding its creation. But political memories are short so that the myth-makers have been able to gull us into the belief that before 5th July 1948 health care in Britain was a scene of chaos and despair and that after that magic date, thanks to Aneurin Bevan's victory over the Conservative Party in unholy alliance with the medical profession and the forces of reaction generally, we made a breakthrough in our pilgrimage to the new Jerusalem. In his hagiography of Bevan, Michael Foot hailed the NHS as "the greatest socialist achievement of the Labour Government."[1]

The part of the myth which has it that only Labour wanted a comprehensive national health service had taken very deep root so that it is now sincerely believed even by those who ought to know better. This was brought home to me very powerfully by an episode which occurred in early December, 1987. In recent years St Thomas' Hospital in London has felt particularly ill-used by the NHS and staff have taken to exploiting the fact that they work just across Westminster Bridge to come regularly to Parliament to air their grievances. As the campaign against the Government's funding of the NHS built up, the doctors and nurses of St Thomas' were determined that they would not be left out and on the afternoon in question about one hundred of them held a meeting in the Grand Committee Room in the Palace of Westminster to which they invited all Members. The meeting was chaired by Stuart Holland, the Labour Member for Vauxhall in whose constituency St Thomas' is sited. The other two Parliamentarians who attended were Lord Ennals, who, as David Ennals, had been Minister of Health in the Labour Government of the 1970s, and myself.

With considerable courtesy, Stuart Holland invited me to speak first. I said I was really there to listen but outlined very briefly the main themes of this book — that whilst government spending on health was high, we should be spending much more *as a nation* but that would mean finding a different structure from the one sustained by both Labour and Conservative Parties since 1948. David Ennals was deeply disturbed by what I had to say and insisted that it was only his Party that had ever wanted a national health service. Ennals is a decent and honourable man with a lot of experience in the health field. He certainly should have known that he was talking nonsense. It was a good demonstration of how powerful and important the myth is to Labour supporters.

Reality was different. For years before 1948 there had been broad general agreement across the political parties on what was needed to improve the nation's health services, a point regularly made during the passage through Parliament of the National Health Service Bill. During the Lords' Debate, for example, a Government spokesman said the Bill was "not the product of any single party or any single Government. It is in fact the outcome of a concerted effort, extending over a long period of years, and involving doctors, laymen and Government, to improve the efficiency of our medical services, and to make them more easily accessible to the public ... Responsible people were advocating a much wider and more comprehensive service long before this ..."[2]

Nor did all-party agreement on the need for change imply that the existing services were universally and gravely deficient. The first chapter of the White Paper on the proposed National Health Service produced by the wartime Coalition Government in 1944 and received with wide acclaim, began thus: "The record of this country in the health and medical services is a good one. The resistance of people to the wear and tear of four years of the Second World War bears testimony to it. Achievements before the war — in lower mortality rates, in the gradual decline of many of the more serious diseases, in safer motherhood and healthier childhood, and generally in the prospect of a longer and healthier life — all substantiate it. There is no question of having to abandon bad services and start afresh. Reform in this field is not a matter of making good what is bad, but of making better what is good already."[3]

In fact — to take just one indicator — it turned out that *infant mortality fell more in the six years before the introduction of the NHS than in the six years afterwards.*

The idea of a comprehensive national health service — although not necessarily one on the lines which emerged in 1948 — had been germinating for at least the previous thirty years; indeed the concept of a national role in the provision of health services had been mooted some four centuries earlier, during the reign of the first Queen Elizabeth and her Poor Law. In 1911, the Royal Commission on the Poor Laws and Relief of Distress having reported its findings two years earlier, Lloyd George brought forward his National Health Insurance Bill. This was designed to remedy the situation in which many people who became ill were thrown onto the poor law. It was not a scheme of medical care as such but constituted an attack on poverty by providing cash payments during absence from work caused by sickness. A small "medical benefit" was allied to these payments to provide for a minimum level of medical care.

Not surprisingly for the period, Lloyd George's NHI scheme was restricted to manual workers and to those non-manual workers with incomes of less than £160 a year in 1911 — a limit which had been raised to £420 by 1948. It did not cover dependants but only the wage-earner, who became entitled to treatment by a "panel doctor", to basic medicines and to sanatorium treatment in cases of tuberculosis. The doctor received a fixed fee for every person on his list as part of a general agreement on remuneration and terms of service negotiated nationally by the medical profession. Uniform controls were placed on chemists' prescription fees and prices.

During 1912 and 1913 Lloyd George's proposals were fiercely resisted by the medical profession. Strongest opposition came from the general practitioners, led by the British Medical Association, but they were also criticised by the hospitals. The British Hospitals Association told Lloyd George that they feared that his legislation would lead to an increase in the demand for in-patient care but reduce subscriptions to the hospitals because henceforth employers would be paying part of the cost of the general practitioner service.

Gradually, however, most doctors came to regard Lloyd George's proposals as inevitable and even desirable — and they were generally welcomed by the public as a step in the right direction. Pressure quickly built up for them to be taken further so that in 1914 Parliament voted funds to include out-patient consultant and specialist treatment within the scope of the NHI scheme. It was still considered that in-patient treatment would be both too costly for the NHI budget and unsuited to an insurance-based system as it would imply a guarantee of hospital treatment when, in practice, admission to hospital might not be possible. Regrettably, the outbreak of war made it necessary to suspend the proposal to extend NHI cover to out-patient treatment.

Even during the war, however, there was a growing consensus that, once peace was restored, further improvement was needed in the scope of national health care. Early in 1917 a Ministry of Reconstruction was set to work to plan the post-war future. It established the Haldane Committee to reorganise the machinery of central government and among the early recommendations of the Committee was a proposal for the creation of a Ministry of Health for England and Wales, which was to take over the many health responsibilties which had accreted to the Local Government Board over the years, to the NHI Commissions for the two countries and to various other government departments.

The Ministry of Health Bill was introduced into Parliament four days before the war ended in 1918 and the Ministry itself came into being on 1st July 1919. The first Minister was Dr Christopher

Addison, formerly Minister of Reconstruction, who had been a distinguished medical academic before entering politics as a Liberal MP.

Addison immediately appointed a Consultative Council on Medical and Allied Services with the future Lord Dawson of Penn as its Chairman and in October 1919 charged it to: "consider and make recommendations as to the scheme or schemes prerequisite for the systematised provision of such forms of medical and allied services as should in the opinion of the Council be available to the inhabitants of a given area."

The composition of the Council, the nature of its recommendations in response to Addison's remit and the speed with which it reached them all demonstrate how opinion had moved during the second decade of the century. Fifteen of the twenty members of the Council came directly from the medical profession and in general their approach contrasted significantly with the pre-war opposition to the NHI arrangements. By now the medical profession had come not only to accept but to be enthusiastic about the scheme. Thus by 1922 the BMA was calling for the income limit for eligibility to the NHI to be raised to £200 a year and for workers' dependants to be brought within its scope. They also called for the coordination of existing health and medical services under some form of health authority.

Working with remarkable despatch, Dawson's Council produced its "Interim Report" by May 1920. In the words of John Pater in his excellent study, *The Making of the National Health Service*, "what they had produced was, in fact, nothing less than the outline of a National Health Service; and in doing so, they laid down the main principles and raised the main issues which governed the pattern of discussion for nearly thirty years."[4]

Lord Dawson and his colleagues insisted on the creation of services which would be available to everyone, although not necessarily free of charge. They were to be founded on the domiciliary services provided by general practitioners, pharmacists, nurses, midwives and health visitors, but should also extend to hospital care. Spotlighting an area where, nearly seventy years on,

Britain still has a sad story to tell, they emphasised the importance of *preventive* medicine and, as part of it, the need for "physical culture" for all. In the first instance this was to be one of the responsibilities of the general practitioner.

The primary health centre was to be a cottage hospital providing a base for domiciliary services such as maternity and child welfare, school health, out-patient and specialist clinics, a dental surgery and an ambulance station. The secondary health centres would be what have now come to be known as district general hospitals, staffed by consultants and specialists, to whom the general practitioners would refer their patients. The consultants would be appointed by a committee representing the hospital, the doctors of the area, the local health authority and the appropriate medical schools. They would be permitted to admit and charge their own private patients and would be paid, on a time basis, for the proportion of the time they spent on patients in the public wards.

Completing the Council proposals were the "supplementary" services regarded as needing separate solutions, such as tuberculosis sanitoria, convalescent homes, mental hospitals, orthopaedic centres and fever hospitals and — at the apex of the system — the teaching hospitals and their medical schools.

Dawson and his colleagues displayed great foresight and a clear understanding of problems which today are very far from being resolved. They pointed the way to solutions which were not adopted but which could still provide us with the answers we have yet to find.

We now have, for example, serious problems of demarcation and financial responsibility between a complex of agencies in the health field, such as the District Health Authorities, the Family Practitioner Committees, the Social Services Departments of the local authorities and the Social Security Offices of the DHSS. Co-ordination and funding arrangements between these bodies remain very unsatisfactory. Dawson's Council proposed that a single health authority should be charged with administering all the services within an (undefined) area. They suggested that three-fifths of the members of these authorities should be locally elected and that two-fifths should be professionals, the majority of them doctors. Each area was also to have a local medical advisory council of ten to twenty members, elected by the local doctors, with the Principal Medical Officer and his two chief assistants as *ex officio* members.

The great problem of exactly how to fund the services was left open, although the Report clearly assumed that the NHI scheme, which had then already been in existence for seven years, could simply be expanded to meet the cost of the domiciliary services. Although some members of the Council advocated free hospital treatment, the majority came down in favour of covering hospital charges by some method of insurance. Nearly seventy years later, when ordinary people are so much better off than they were then, I am sure this is an idea we must now look at again — just as we must re-examine the organisational and funding arrangements of the health service. What we now have, after forty years of constant modification of the superstructure of the NHS, is a system which encumbers Ministers with total accountability for virtually everything that happens throughout the entire service and yet leaves them with very little power. This is an arrangement which is both ludicrous in itself and also a classic recipe for organisational and political disaster.

The Dawson Report could have initiated a national debate on how to provide and fund health care in Britain which might well have produced answers very different from those which emerged in the National Health Service Act over a quarter of a century later. Tragically, however, the debate was quickly stifled — even though the significance of the Report was immediately recognised. The *British Medical Journal*, for example, observed that "its implementation would have a profound effect on the future of medicine in England" and *The Hospital* said "it was of transcendent importance but that its proposals would be costly and its implementation would inevitably entail the disappearance of the voluntary hospital system, as then known".[5] The controversial issues raised by the Dawson proposals — the problems of funding, control and local responsibilities (*plus ca change!*) — proved too difficult to handle and the economic blizzard which hit the country soon after the Report was published finally ensured that it was buried.

It had been written in the spirit which had created the Ministry of Reconstruction in 1917, showing a readiness to think boldly and imaginatively in order to create services which measured up to the needs of "a land fit for heroes". But the budget crisis developed so quickly and so acutely, that only nine months after the publication of the Interim Report of Dawson's Council, the Ministry of Health was urging on local authorities the need for "rigid economies of public resources". All thought of fundamental change or of the expansion of medical services had therefore to be postponed. In essence, it remained suspended throughout the between-the-wars years of depression and overseas menace.

Even under these shadows, however, some progress was made especially in the hospital sector.

By 1914 the voluntary hospitals provided nearly all of the facilities for acute medical and surgical care throughout the country. However the war had seriously hit the income of these hospitals and therefore in January 1921 Addison set up a Committee under the chairmanship of Lord Cave to recommend ways of improving their finances. The Cave Committee accepted that the voluntary hospitals, of which at that time there were 845 with 44,000 beds in England and Wales, needed financial help from public funds but insisted that it should be not only strictly limited but also temporary. They believed that to arrange for continued public financial support would undermine the voluntary system by causing voluntary contributions to dry up, which would in turn create a need for the direct public provision of hospitals themselves and that these would be much more expensive to operate.

The Government did not accept all the funding proposals made by the Cave Committee but agreed to provide £500,000 for maintenance support. In the event, this sum — very small even by the standards of the time — proved to be sufficient for the purpose. The incomes of the voluntary hospitals recovered more quickly than had been anticipated and a system of contributory schemes advocated by the Cave Committee proved to be so popular that the financial situation of the hospitals was transformed. Under these schemes wage earners made weekly payments to the hospitals, supplemented by contributions from their employers.

Long before the system of voluntary hospitals had emerged Britain had already developed a network of Poor Law hospitals operated by the local authorities. These institutions were unpopular, both because of their nature and the stigma still attaching to them but also because of the generally low standard of care that they provided. After his appointment as Minister of Health in 1924, the Conservative Neville Chamberlain became very concerned that there were thousands of empty beds in public hospitals whilst there were long queues waiting for admission to the voluntary hospitals. During the years of his tenure he emphasised the urgency of the need to improve co-operation between the two hospital systems but encountered great resistance. Among the large body of people who were convinced of the superiority of voluntary hospitals were many who believed, unjustifiably, that Chamberlain wished to bring them into state control. There was much fear about the threat of a state medical service with salaried doctors.

Chamberlain's repeated calls therefore went largely unheeded at the time but the Local Government Act of 1929 opened the way for improvement in the standard of public hospitals. It transferred to local authorities all the responsibilities of the Poor Law Board of Guardians and allowed the authorities to provide the full range of hospital treatment. The hospital provisions of the Act were not made compulsory and their implementation was undoubtedly delayed by the economic and political crisis of 1931 and by the Depression which continued thereafter. However, throughout the 1930s a network of public hospitals began to develop, all the more so as the "Poor Law" stigma slowly wore off.

The real stimulus needed to promote the co-operation between voluntary and public hospitals advocated by Chamberlain came in 1938 with the recognition that war was imminent and from the understanding gained from the Spanish Civil War of the scale of casualties that could be inflicted on civilians by bombing raids. The first survey of hospitals in England and Wales since 1863 revealed that voluntary hospitals provided some 78,000 beds and that local authorities controlled a further 320,000, some 150,000 of which were in mental institutions and 35,000 in isolation hospitals and tuberculosis sanatoria.

The Government accordingly established an Emergency Medical Service (originally known as the Emergency Hospital Scheme) under which the Ministry of Health became responsible for the treatment of casualties and thus, for the first time, was empowered to decide the role each hospital would play. Although the existing local government and hospital authorities provided a regional framework, in a manner and at a speed that would have been unthinkable without the war emergency, the Ministry found itself in a position of control and leadership to which it had not previously even aspired and which few had sought on its behalf.

As the war went on the EMS developed into something very much more than a service only for civilian casualties and for the sick and wounded members of the armed forces. Through running it, the Ministry became closely involved in undertaking a huge expansion of pathology, blood transfusion, pharmacy and rehabilitation services and also in deciding the salaries of nurses and other staff, in organising and providing catering services and ambulances.

Thus the foundation of the post-war National Health Service had already been comprehensively laid and indeed it was a Conservative Minister, Walter Elliott, who in the very first months of the war already raised the question of whether the EMS should not be turned into a permanent state hospital service.

The Planning Begins

By the end of the 1930's there was a wide spectrum of agreement on the need to develop a national system of health care and there is a good deal of evidence which, as Rudolf Klein points out in *The Politics of the National Health Service*, "shows civil servants taking the initiative in generating policy options unprompted, as far as can be judged from the records, by the politicians."[6] Klein notes that in 1938 the then Permanent Secretary to the Health Ministry, Sir John Maude, set up a small group of civil servants to consider the future of the health services. At its first meeting Maude outlined two possible lines of approach: "either the gradual extension of National Health Insurance to further classes of the community and by new statutory benefits, or the gradual development of the local authority services."

On 21st September 1939, another member of the group, Sir Arthur MacNalty, Chief Medical Officer for the Ministry, put forward a third option: "the suggestion that the hospitals of England and Wales should be administered as a national hospital service by the Ministry."

This turned out to be a crucial document amongst those that led health care in Britain away from paths which would almost certainly have produced better results for the vast majority of us and which, without any doubt, would also have made life easier (not meaning merely more comfortable) for governments. Locally funded regional services — the solution adopted by a number of countries — would at least have gone a very long way towards removing the issue of health from the party political battlefield where in this country it now features so prominently — and unproductively. To have developed Sir John Maude's national health insurance approach would have left open the possibility of grafting on and growing towards, without much difficulty, a system of personal health insurance which would have produced not only the extra funding now so desperately needed by the NHS but which could still make Britain's health care arrangements the best in the world.

But these were not the roads chosen. Instead, the National Health Service emerged in 1948 on lines very close to those set out by Sir Arthur MacNalty in 1939.

MacNalty came down in favour of "nationalising" the hospitals whilst recognising the difficulties and arguments that would be advanced against it. One of the objections was that it would "dry up the flow of voluntary subscriptions which largely contribute to relieving the ratepayer and the taxpayer of the cost of hospital provision." Second: "the majority of the medical profession would be bitterly opposed to it. This would cause much dissension, controversy and ill feeling at a time when it is vitally important that national unity should be preserved." Third: the proposal implied "a radical change in the policy of the Ministry. Hitherto we have always worked on the assumption that the Ministry of Health was an advisory, supervisory and subsidising department that had no direct executive function." Lastly, "from the point of view of local authorities, executive control of all hospitals by the State might excite opposition and present difficulties."[7]

All these arguments were, indeed, heard in the debate on the proposals for the NHS in the immediate post-war years but, as MacNalty had already foreseen in 1939, the operation and development of the EMS persuaded most people that nationalisation would provide the right answer.

The next milestone signalling the emergence of a broad national consensus on health came in 1942 with the publication by Sir William Beveridge of his *Report on Social Insurance and Allied Services*. For our purposes the real significance of the famous Report is how *little* it says about the post-war structure of health care. Beveridge stated that "from the standpoint of social security, a health service providing full preventive and curative treatment of every kind to every citizen without exceptions, without remuneration limit and without an economic barrier at any point to delay recourse to it, is the ideal plan."[8] His plan assumed ("Assumption B") "the establishment of comprehensive health and rehabilitation services providing treatment for all citizens without a charge on treatment"[9] but he made it clear "that no final detailed proposals, even as to the financial basis" of these services could be included in his Report.

Thus there was nothing in Beveridge's *opus* which established that the health service which was to form such a crucial element in the "welfare state" and "cradle to the grave" security could *only* be provided in the form which finally emerged in 1948 and which thereafter has been held to be sacrosanct. Beveridge's health objectives could have been — and could still be — achieved by other means, almost certainly more effectively. Indeed Beveridge was a strong believer in the insurance principle, declaring that "benefit in return for contributions, rather than free allowances from the state, is what the people of Britain desire". He was in favour of "establishing a national minimum" which "should leave room and encouragement for voluntary action by each individual to provide more than the minimum for himself and his family." He also believed that "it is reasonable that insured persons should contribute something for such services" as surgical appliances, convalescent homes and nursing and, in some cases, the "hotel expenses" of a stay in hospital.

Beveridge looked forward to the creation of a health service which would "diminish disease by prevention and cure" and thus ease the burden of social security payments which the implementation of his proposals would entail.[10]

In 1943 the Coalition Government announced that it accepted the need for a comprehensive health scheme and set in hand the work necessary to hammer out the details. These emerged in the 1944 White Paper which was presented to Parliament by the Conservative Minister of Health, Henry Willink, where it was greeted with a wide measure of approval. This was despite the fact that it was a compromise document seeking to reconcile many interests — local authorities, voluntary hospitals, hospital consultants, general practitioners, the advocates of a salaried medical service and others. In the words of Harry Eckstein in his study, *The English Health Service*: "Very few announcements of public policy have had a more enthusiastic Parliamentary reception. Speech after speech welcomed the White Paper's proposals and congratulated the Minister for producing them. The only sour note of the session that was otherwise all sweetness and light was struck by certain spokesmen on the medical left who thought the proposals were not sufficiently unequivocal in their commitment to a free National Health Service and a few spokesmen of the medical right who were worried about the implications rather than the actual proposals for the scheme. But the Parliamentary chorus lay somewhere between the enthusiastic soprano of Dr Edith

Summerskill and the gloomy bass of Sir Ernest Graham Little.
The White Paper was overwhelmingly approved."[11]

The White Paper, which had been written by Sir John Horton,
future Permanent Secretary to the Ministry of Health, was founded
on two principles which were accepted on all sides by 1944 and
which were to remain the foundation of the National Health
Service when it finally emerged. First, the service was to be
comprehensive so that "in future every man, woman and child can
rely on getting all the advice and treatment and care which they may
need in matters of personal health; that what they get shall be the
best medical and other facilities available." The second principle
was that the service should be "free" so "that their getting these
shall not depend on whether they can pay for them, or any other
factor irrelevant to the real need — the real need being to bring the
country's full resources to bear upon reducing ill health and
promoting good health in all its citizens."[12]

It was envisaged that the cost of this "free" service would be met
out of taxation and out of local rates, possibly supplemented a little
by insurance payments, and that the total charge to the public
funds would be some £132 million. Thus Horton's figure was even
lower than the £170 million which had been Beveridge's estimate, as
it was expected that under the White Paper proposals a
considerable amount of private practice and voluntary contributions would continue. In the event, total expenditure on
Bevan's version of the Health Service in England and Wales in the
first year of its operation turned out to be £339,600,000.

The White Paper recognised "certain danger in making personal
health the subject of a national service at all. It is the danger of over-
organisation ..." The solution proposed was that the Minister
should have responsibility for planning the service but that
executive responsibility should be vested in local organisations —
new joint authorities which would probably comprise the counties
and county boroughs. These authorities would be directly
responsible for running the hospital and consultant services whilst
responsibility for local clinics and other personal social services
would remain with the existing councils. The voluntary hospitals

would be linked with the system by their entering into a contractual relationship with the joint authorities "for the performance of agreed services."[13]

Public accountability was to be achieved by ensuring that "effective decisions on policy must lie entirely with elected representatives answerable to the people for the decisions they take." In other words, these people were to be the local government councillors serving on the joint authorities. The White Paper, however, also recognised a need that might conflict with this, of medical professionals taking part in decision-making. It therefore proposed a Central Health Services Council to advise on national policy, with parallel bodies at the local level. General practitioners would, if they wished, be able to keep their independent status, receiving a capitation fee for each patient, but the Central Medical Board would be empowered to control the distribution of doctors around the country. General practitioners would be encouraged to group themselves in health centres provided by the joint authorities but under contract to the Central Medical Board.

Despite the warmth of the initial reception of the White Paper, opposition to it began to develop quickly from a number of quarters. Local authorities, although relieved that the danger of outright nationalisation appeared to have been averted, were dissatisfied at the prospect of the new joint authorities taking over their hospitals. The voluntary hospitals believed that, whilst nominally providing for their continued independence, the scheme would deprive them of vital patients' income and would be, in the words of Henry Willink to the War Cabinet's Reconstruction Committee, "a mortal blow". Those on the left grumbled that the move towards a salaried medical service should go much further.

Fiercest of all, however, was the hostility which flared up from the medical profession. Writing in the *British Medical Journal*, one correspondent charged that "the ultimate intention of the proposals is brilliantly camouflaged ... Underlying the subtle phrases of the White Paper is the mailed fist of bureaucratic control carefully wrapped up in the velvet glove of political diplomacy."

The leader in the same issue took a similar line: "It is important to recognise the unmistakable direction in which the mind of the Government is moving — and that is towards the institution of a whole-time salaried medical service, with the proviso that ... private practice should not be denied to those who want it and that doctors in the public service may provide it ... It is difficult to see how, in the kind of evolutionary changes which are so persuasively outlined, private practice as we know it today can survive as much more than a shadow of itself."[14]

In June 1945 Henry Willink brought back to the Cabinet a revised set of proposals which aimed to modify "certain features in the original plan which had been unpopular with the local authorities, voluntary hospitals and the medical profession."

But, just a few weeks later, he and the rest of the Conservative Ministers were swept from office by Labour's landslide victory in the General Election. The spirit engendered by that event is well captured by Michael Foot in the opening sentences of the second volume of his book on Aneurin Bevan: "No socialist who saw it will forget the blissful dawn of July 1945. The great war in Europe had ended; the lesser war in Asia might be ending soon. This background to the scene in Britain naturally deepened the sense of release and breathtaking opportunity ... When the scale of the Labour Party's victory became known on the night of 26th July, bonfires were lit, people danced in the streets and young and old crowded into halls all over the country to acclaim their elected standard-bearers ..."[15]

And the elected standard-bearer appointed to carry Britain's health care into the new socialist Utopia was Aneurin Bevan, Churchill's back-bench scourge of the war years. Some of the mystique which has developed around the National Health Service had its origin in the personality of Bevan himself, a brilliant but erratic figure of the romantic left. Attlee might well have chosen a colleague like Morrison, Cripps or Dalton for his Minister of Health. The portfolio was, after all, an important part of his government's programme. Any one of them would have brought a more realistic and workmanlike approach to the task than did

Bevan. But none of them would have been able to envelop the whole enterprise so effectively with his own personal aura.

Thus the National Health Service became entangled with the very name of Aneurin Bevan. Yet the reality was that the organisation which emerged after two years of his labours represented no more than a staging-point on the continuum which had been developing since at least as early as 1920. As Rudolf Klein observes: "In a sense the virulent hostility of Bevan's critics — both on the Conservative benches in Parliament and among the medical profession — flattered his achievement and exaggerated the extent to which he broke with the sedimentary consensus that had been built up over the preceding years."[16]

3
Bevan's Bill

The National Health Service Bill which Bevan introduced in March 1946 differed in only one significant respect from the amended version of the 1944 proposals which the Coalition Government had agreed on some nine months earlier. Bevan rejected Willink's scheme for the hospitals and reverted to the clear-cut nationalisation of the hospital service which Sir Arthur MacNalty had proposed in September 1939. The apparent success of the Emergency Medical Service in the seven years after 1939 reinforced his ideological confidence that nationalisation would work.

The inevitable consequence of this step was, in the words of Bevan's Cabinet memorandum of 5th October 1945, "the centralising of the whole finance of the country's hospital system, taking it right out of local rating and government."[1] The memorandum was considered by the Labour Cabinet on 11th October and received a very mixed welcome. Bevan failed to carry several of his powerful colleagues. Hugh Dalton, the Chancellor of the Exchequer, reserved his position, Arthur Greenwood feared the plan was too radical and Herbert Morrison, Lord President of the Council, was strongly opposed.

Bevan did recognise at least some of the dangers which worried his critics. Responding to Morrison's warning that the scheme would produce bureaucratic over-centralisation, he wrote: "A centralised service must indeed be planned so as to avoid rigidity. That is why I have proposed that the hospital service shall be administered locally by regional boards and district committees . . . it is precisely by the selection of the right men and women to serve on these bodies that I hope to be able to give them substantial executive powers, subject to a broad financial control and so prevent rigidity." But he went on: "Admittedly, this is a field in which there is room for development in the techniques of government but the problems that will arise should not be incapable of solution."[2]

He was wrong. The problems created by Bevan's blueprint for the NHS have for forty years resisted all attempts at solution so that they are now more insoluble — and give rise to more bitterness and frustration — than ever.

Complaints were also heard from Labour's backbenches. Mr (later Sir) Frederick Messer, MP for South Tottenham, for example, whilst acknowledging that the Bill made "a very big step forward", expressed some trenchant criticisms in his speech in the Second Reading debate. He charged that it was a medical service rather than a health service Bill, offering little for preventive health care and nothing at all for after-care and rehabilitation. Messer pointed out that the proposals were not comprehensive, would not create a unified health service encompassing areas such as child welfare, district nursing and dental care and were, moreover, not democratic. He asked why, in creating the regional boards, Bevan had "lost faith in the elected principle."

Particularly noteworthy, especially given the subsequent near-canonisation of Bevan as founder of the NHS and the sanctification of the NHS itself as the purest expression of socialism in action, is that, in making his proposals, he largely ignored the established policy of the Labour Party. In April 1943 the Party had published *National Service for Health* in which it had proposed the creation of elected regional committees for all local government purposes, with a health committee to plan the health service for the region. Labour's Conference held in Blackpool in 1944 had endorsed Willink's White Paper and had demanded that local authorities be given control over municipal hospitals and medical services.

To look back over the years as I have had the pleasure of doing in preparing this book is to discover a political fairy tale which has surely been sold more effectively than any other in our history. Although I came into politics only in 1978, I like to think of myself as reasonably politically aware and with some knowledge of our past — and certainly not as one of the more gullible targets for Labour Party propaganda. Yet it was surprising to discover the extent to which even someone with my sort of background has come to accept the carefully-cultivated legend that, in the heroic battle for the creation of the National Health Service, the brilliant Bevan led a united Labour Party to victory over ferocious Conservative opposition.

It is true that the Conservative Party voted against the Second Reading of the Bill (probably an error of political tactics) and — like a number of Labour Ministers and backbenchers — had reservations about various aspects of it. Nevertheless, the Conservatives had consistently supported the principles on which it was based, as they had regularly demonstrated during their years in office.

The Conservative Health spokesman, Richard Law, spelled out his Party's position during the Second Reading debate: "I am anxious to make clear our positions on these benches in regard to the principle of the national, comprehensive, 100% health service. Of course we accept that principle today, as we accepted it in 1944, when the Coalition White Paper was published. I assure the Minister that on this side of the House we are just as anxious as he is, or any of his Hon. or Rt. Hon. Friends, by his side or behind him are, to give the people of this country the fullest possible benefits which can come from the acceptance of the principle of the comprehensive health service. I hope that the Minister will understand that. We accept the principle and we accept the consequences that flow from it. We understand, for example, that once we are committed, as we are gladly committed, to the principle of a 100% service we require an enormous expansion and development of the health services as a whole. We understand, once we accept the principle, that we are committed to a far greater degree of co-ordination, or planning as it is usually called, than we have ever known before."

Law emphasised the degree of consensus and continuity which existed on the need to reform the structure of health care. He referred to the work of his colleague, Henry Willink, as Health Minister in the Coalition Government and said that: "... had the General Election gone the other way, I do not doubt that he would have introduced, before this, a Bill which would have differed from this Bill only in that my Rt Honourable and Learned Friend would not have attempted to control, own and direct the hospital service of this country or to interfere with that age-old relationship which exists, always has existed and in our view ought to continue to exist, between a doctor and his patient."[3]

The Conservative aversion for the proposal to nationalise hospitals that Bevan had now resurrected was shared by many in the ranks of the Labour Party. Acceptance of the proposal was, indeed, a sudden *volte face* by the Government itself. On 15th February 1946, just five weeks before Bevan's Bill was published, Herbert Morrison was still telling the House that: "... the view of the Minister of Health and the Government was that it would not be right to take the hospitals over into a national concern. I think that is quite right ..."[4]

Writing now, at a time when Bevan's nationalisation of Britain's hospitals has for so long been regarded on all sides as the Ark of the Covenant, immutable and unchallengeable, it is — to put it at its mildest — ironic to consider that his proposal had been strongly challenged by his Cabinet colleagues, went completely against the published policies of the Labour Party and was opposed by the local authorities and the great majority of the medical profession.

What ensured Bevan's canonisation was the unfortunate nature of the resistance of the doctors to his proposals. Not all the details of their lengthy and noisy struggles against the Minister need be re-told here but they do prompt one or two reflections on the way the medical profession has sometimes chosen to wage political warfare in a manner that has defeated its own interests. Certain lessons can be drawn which are relevant today as we search for ways to revitalise health care. No trade union or any other sectional interest has ever come near the British Medical Association in the conspicuous ferocity and easily exposable guile with which it has pursued its ends.

As we noted earlier, the doctors waged a determined battle against the National Health Insurance Act of Lloyd George in 1911. As the Act took effect they came to understand that its provisions improved the income and employment prospects of the medical profession and so, within two years, they were pressing strongly for its extension. From 1945 until the inception of the National Health Service on the "Appointed Day" of 5th July 1948, they conducted a remarkable campaign against many of the changes which had for so long been under consideration. Yet it was only a few years after the "surrender" that they came to realise that they had, in fact, wrested a good deal from Bevan if a "good deal" meant security of employment on incomes that appeared fairly high for the foreseeable future.* From motives which were a mixture of altruism and self-interest — an entirely normal human pheno- menon — the great majority of doctors soon became strongly committed defenders of the new regime. This tendency was reinforced as the BMA began to develop techniques which were much better designed than their earlier efforts to generate the pressure on politicians which was necessary to persuade them to pass over increasing quantities of public resources to health care, whilst effectively resisting many attempts to exercise sensible control over their own use of those resources.

This record gives reason to hope that the political leaders of the profession, who have been shown by no means always to be in step with their colleagues, will be fiercely resistant to any new thinking on how to provide better health care in Britain — but that the resistance will be short-lived. Once any new system is in operation and can be seen to benefit doctors as well as improve the quality of health care, they will become its most committed and passionate defenders.

The profession does not, of course, always speak with a single voice or have a single set of interests. In particular, doctors in

* Bevan said later he had "... stuffed the doctors' mouths with pound notes."

general practice, who are dominant in the BMA, tend to be divided from those who are specialists and consultants in hospitals, whose views are usually represented by the leaders of what are known as the Royal Colleges. This division, which is much sharper in medicine in Britain than in other countries, was as much a reality in 1946 as it is today and Bevan was able to take some advantage of it in his battle with the profession. Thus in the spring of 1948, when it appeared likely that the BMA would take action to frustrate the introduction of the NHS on the Appointed Day, the Presidents of the Royal Colleges intervened to reach an accommodation. Commenting on this incident, Harry Eckstein has noted: "Some have alleged that the Presidents took a conciliatory attitude because Bevan had "bribed" the specialists with financial and administrative concessions, promising large incomes and independence of teaching hospitals from the other hospital authorities about to be created. This is plausible, for the service, as finally constituted, does in fact favour specialists from teaching hospitals but more plausible is the view that specialists were favourably disposed towards the service from the start."[5]

Wherever the truth may lie, the fact is that the specialists did win some notable concessions from Bevan. Teaching hospitals, on which they depended for their eminence (and, in many cases, high incomes) were given special status, with their own governing bodies directly under the Ministry of Health. They were allowed to retain private pay beds in NHS hospitals, in the teeth of opposition from much of the Labour Party. A new system of merit awards for hospital consultants was introduced.

Yet the general practitioners, too, came away from their battles with Aneurin Bevan far from empty-handed. Whilst he insisted on ending the system of the sale and purchase of practices, offering £66 million in compensation (equivalent to about £780 million in 1987 prices), he made many concessions. The 1944 White Paper had opened up the prospect of a national corps of doctors directly employed by the Central Medical Board. In the face of strong objections from the doctors, the Conservatives had abandoned this idea in favour of Insurance Committees involving the local authorities. Bevan went further by agreeing that general practitioners should have contracts with local executive committees, on which there would be a greater representation of the medical profession than under previous arrangements, thus removing any threat that doctors would become either civil servants or local authority employees.

By April 1948, with the Appointed Day only three months away and facing a very serious challenge from the BMA, Bevan had made a still greater concession. He went to the House and undertook to bring in an Amending Bill to make impossible the introduction of a whole-time salaried service under the NHS Act or any subsequent regulations. The objective of a salaried service was strongly supported within the ranks of the Labour Party.

The most important gain of all for the medical profession, however, flowed directly from Bevan's abandonment of the concept that health services at the regional level should be in the hands of the elected representatives of the local authorities. This concession made it possible for doctors *qua* doctors to serve on the new regional and district authorities, something for which the medical profession had long fought. Bevan took up this idea with enthusiasm early in the battle. In his memorandum to Cabinet in October 1945, for example, he insisted: "The full principle of direct public responsibility must, of course, be maintained, but we can — and must — afford to bring the voice of the expert right into direct participation of the planning and running of the service."[6]

The doctors had good reason to be satisfied — and Bevan made it clear that he was not prepared to bestow the same favours on other workers in the health service. When the TUC General Secretary, Sir Walter Citrine, raised the question, Bevan responded that no-one else would be on regional boards or hospital management committees in any capacity that represented their occupation. Rejecting the idea of such participation, he said; "If the nurses were to be consulted, why not also the hospital domestics? The radiotherapists? The physiotherapists? And so on."[7]

Looking back over the welter of debate that attended the birth of the health service, from the perspective offered forty years on, it is surprising to discover the issues which were *not* discussed. Apart from the particular matters raised with such vigour by the medical profession, the rest of the debate was almost entirely centred on relatively minor administrative and technical alternatives to an agreed objective. For years a consensus had been developing across the political parties that there could and should be a National Health Service which was both free and comprehensive. No-one seems to have been prepared to point to the possibility that the demand for "free" medical care might always expand at a much greater rate than the country would be able or willing to provide. And no-one considered opportunity costs — the benefits which alternative uses of the same resources might bring. Indeed the view that as the nation grew healthier as the result of the better services provided, real demand would actually fall was widely-held. Twenty years later, having served his turn as Minister of Health, Enoch Powell was to describe this view as "a miscalculation of sublime proportions".

Yet ten years on from the Appointed Day, in a House of Commons debate to mark the anniversary of the NHS, it was still a belief held by the then Conservative Minister of Health despite a decade of experience showing it was wrong. On 30th July 1958, Derek Walker-Smith told the House: "We have to aim at the prevention and, where possible, the elimination of illness, resulting in a positive improvement in health, reflected in the factory, the foundry and the farm and not merely in the convalescent homes. If we do this, better health will go hand in hand with diminished costs (*sic*) and we shall be able successfully to discharge both our social and our economic duty."

This extraordinarily persistent belief seems to show a massive misunderstanding of human nature and the need for close and conspicuous connections between the services performed and rewards received.

It is perhaps not surprising, therefore, that in all the debates and studies the resources that would be needed were not seriously examined, nor was attention given to the ways in which demand would grow in the ensuing years. The blandness (a less charitable word would be irresponsibility) of this approach was epitomised by Bevan himself in moving the Second Reading of his Bill in the Commons: "It has been the firm conclusion of all parties that money ought not to be permitted to stand in the way of obtaining an efficient health service".[8]

Much painful experience has now taught all of us that, in seeking an effective system of health care, the question of resources cannot be so blithely disregarded.

The way Britain slipped into broad acceptance of the NHS formula as the only system of delivering a satisfactory level of health care to the nation seems in retrospect to indicate a mixture of blindness and ill-justified optimism. It was the *zeitgeist* of Bloomsbury which also led us into the quicksands of neo-Keynesianism from which, since 1979, we have made a painful but increasingly successful escape. The failure to foresee how pressures on the service would develop and the belief that whatever the level of demand, resources would somehow be found to meet it, now seems incomprehensible. No doubt the prevalence of this view among British politicians of the day owed a great deal not only to the Bloomsbury approach but also to the euphoria of our victory in war. This had fuelled the belief that when a project was of sufficient importance, even in peacetime conditions the government would always be able to find the necessary resources and that good central planning and administration would ensure that those resources would always be used to optimum affect. It is significant that Germany was spared that euphoria and constructed a very different system of health care.

There was a second factor in the creation of the NHS which has tended to be overlooked, as Aneurin Bevan reminded the House when he spoke in the debate to mark the tenth anniversary of the inauguration of the service on 30 July 1958: "Two main conceptions underlay the National Health Service. The first was to provide a comprehensive, free, health service for all the people of the country at time of need. The second — I shall call particular attention to this later, because it is somewhat overlooked — was the redistribution of national income by a special method of financing the Health Service".[9] There is a saying sometimes used by craftsmen to the effect that a tool designed for two purposes ends up by doing neither of them very well. It is a thought we should keep in mind as we seek to improve on the blueprint of 1948.

After forty years of what has hitherto been effective propaganda about the inherent virtues of the NHS ("which would *still* be the 'envy of the world' if only those stupid politicians in office would only spend enough money on it"), few people now realise how easily we could have adopted a significantly different system of health care after the war, one which would probably have proved much better able to cope with the pressures that have grown and continue to grow so strongly. As we noted earlier, experience in other countries suggests that either regional or, preferably, an insurance-based system would have offered far better possibilities, for example, of increasing the amount we spend, as sensible and responsible individuals, on our own health and that of our families. These alternatives would also have kept the issue of health funding at a greater distance from the unhelpful bear-garden of national politics. Instead, we adopted a structure and a system of funding which, despite all the efforts at improvement over the years, has proved to be tight and rigid. Now that we have reached breaking point, the changes which have become inescapable appear to present enormous political difficulties. Yet the longer we put off the changes, the greater those difficulties seem to be.

In fact I am sure that when, as a nation, we are finally persuaded of the need to steel ourselves to take the fence of NHS reform, that fence will turn out to be lower than it now appears. But I do not underestimate the problems. The 1.2 million people employed in the service and their families are themselves crucial. The fact that we have more doctors and nurses than ever before and that in real terms they are also better paid than ever means that most of them (and certainly those who have become "medical politicians") will fight to the last ditch to preserve the system that they have learned to venerate and, perhaps unconsciously, to *use* so well. They will resist budgetary control, feeling a generalised righteousness that they are "defending" the sacred cause of the health service against insensate calculating machines at the Treasury. They will be powerfully supported by a large section of the middle class, the section of society which has used its skills and position to obtain greatest benefits from the NHS. (Many are successors of those who, in 1948, were earning over £420 a year and were therefore at that time excluded from the provisions of the NHI scheme.)

The most passionate defenders of all, of course, will be the Labour Party for whom, as the years go by, the National Health Service assumes an ever more sacrosanct status. The Party has kept itself going for decades on legends about the achievements of the Attlee government. Yet, one by one, those achievements have turned to ashes. Nationalisation is now seen to have been a disaster in virtually every area in which it was tried. Where industries have been brought back into the private sector almost everyone has benefited: the workers, customers and the national economy. For most people now, nationalisation is personified by Arthur Scargill leading thugs against the police and against ordinary workers who want to work. The powers given to trade unions are now seen seriously to have held back industrial development and therefore employment and to have infringed grossly on personal liberties. People have massively rejected Labour's enthusiasm for council housing and have chosen to own the houses in which they live. Most already now accept that in the post-war years education in Britain — under Butler's 1944 Act — at least took some wrong turnings.

Out of all this wreckage of Labour's political and intellectual heritage, the main item clinging on for survival is its claim — very poorly based, as we have seen — to be the founding and sole father of the National Health Service. It will therefore fight change less like a stag at bay than like a defiant dinosaur defending its last egg.

But those of us who are interested in producing a health system which will be able to cope with the needs of the future rather than defending the mistakes of the past are unlikely to be deterred by the reactionaries.

4

"Cascades of Medicine"

So, after a generation of debate, the great experiment of the National Health Service was finally launched. A centrally controlled and funded system was to be created to deliver medical care free to the whole population. It was a massive collectivist step in a society which was still pluralist and in which, despite all the pressures on it, the mixed economy still survived.

Britain was setting off down a path followed by almost no other democratic country. And as the years went by it was a route which was to remain untrodden by others. The overwhelming majority of Western nations developed health care systems which were founded on principles very different from those finally adopted for the NHS.

Despite the achievements of the service — and no responsible critics of the system would deny that they have been considerable — the weaknesses inherent in the structure which emerged in July 1948 quickly began to show.

Concern began to develop almost immediately about NHS costs — an issue which, as we have seen, had been virtually ignored in most of the debates which had preceded the Appointed Day. The dilemma which had been identified and argued over at length — how to avoid bureaucratisation and reconcile the needs of what is in essence a local service with centralised control — did emerge quickly and resisted all attempts to resolve it in the decades that followed. The same is true of the search for a satisfactory relationship between the medical and other professionals in the service with those responsible for funding and administering it.

In this chapter we look at how spending on the health service has burgeoned over the years, in a manner which starkly demonstrates the fatuity of the view that the NHS would quickly create a healthier nation which would actually begin to reduce its demands on the health services. There could be no better illustration of the perils of the sort of centralised planning that produced the NHS when intelligent and experienced men can fall into such fundamental error.

Only months after the launch of the service, Aneurin Bevan was complaining to Hugh Gaitskell of the "cascades of medicine pouring down British throats." That cascade has continued to increase ever since.

Nor did even Bevan — at least after the Appointed Day — really seem to expect that it would be otherwise. By March 1950 he felt it necessary to spell out to his Cabinet colleagues the realities of the pressures on NHS spending:

> Allowing for all sensible administrative measures to prevent waste, the plain fact is that the cost of the health service not only will, but ought to, increase. Most of the hospitals fall far short of any proper standard; accommodation needs to be increased, particularly for tuberculosis and mental health — indeed some of the mental hospitals are very near to a public scandal and we are lucky that they have not so far attracted more limelight and publicity. Throughout the service there are piling up arrears of essential capital work. Also it is in this field, particularly, that constant new development will always be needed to keep pace with research progress (as, recently, in penicillin, streptomycin, cortisone etc.) and to expand essential specialist services, such as hearing aids or ophthalmic services. The position cannot be evaded that a nationally owned and administered hospital service *will always involve a very considerable and expanding Exchequer outlay,* (my italics). If that possibility cannot, for financial reasons, be faced, then the only alternatives (to my mind thoroughly undesirable), are either to give up — in whole or in part — the idea of national responsibility for the hospitals or also to import into the scheme some regular source of revenue such as the recovery of charges from those who use it. I am afraid it is clear that we cannot have it both ways.[1]

Bevan's forecast proved correct. People have come to believe that they have a right to good health and that the system has the duty and should have the capacity to prolong and improve the quality of their lives. This is, of course, a universal phenomenon and all experience shows that the richer a country becomes, the higher proportion of the national wealth is spent, either by governments or individuals, on health services. One important factor in this growth is that health care is a highly labour intensive activity. The special characteristic of the British system is the unique extent to which demand for more health spending leads directly to increased pressure on the state Exchequer and therefore to ever more political trouble for the Government of the day.

The change in public attitudes brought about by the NHS was brought home to me vividly in the first speech I gave after becoming a Health Minister in September 1985. The Conservative Party Conference, about a fortnight after the reshuffle, was held in Blackpool that year and the Northern Region of the British Medical Association used the opportunity to organise a meeting to which they invited a DHSS Minister. My two senior colleagues declined — one saying he was too busy and the other that he had only just been appointed to the job — but I was happy to accept, seeing it both as a useful part of the learning process I needed and as an opportunity to show the medical profession something of the new Ministerial team. Moreover, I strongly believe, as they used to say in FCO telegrams, that *"les absents ont toujours tort"* — not a maxim always followed by Government Departments and Ministers.

Having mugged up my voluminous Departmental briefing — and having, as usually seemed advisable, thrown away the standard speech which the civil servants had constructed from the memory bank of the Departmental word processor — in my opening talk I duly listed many of the advances achieved in the NHS since 1979. I went through the standard litany of increases in the numbers of doctors, nurses, patients treated and the substantial growth in the amount of the nation's resources devoted to health care, emphasising that this could only continue if we had the benefit of a healthy economy, which in turn, as all experience demonstrated, would only be achieved by Conservative policies (it was, after all, a political speech).

From the beginning, the atmosphere of the meeting was distinctly chilly. The temperature was set by the opening remarks of the Secretary of the BMA, Dr John Havard, who offered an elegant and courteous welcome to the neophyte but which, nevertheless, exuded condescension and a weary recognition that here was yet one more politician that the BMA would have to educate and bring into line. Havard's performance, as I came to realise later, was a classic demonstration of the relationship between the spokesmen of the medical profession and the politicians which has developed over generations. He warned me, for example, that in my new duties I must realise that in their day-to-day contacts with the rest of humanity doctors became accustomed to acting like God and this tended to colour their attitudes. He was not joking. The "God syndrome" of the medical profession is a political factor of considerable importance.

One much favoured technique of speakers facing the prospect of a difficult meeting is to make a very long opening speech, preferably read in a near-monotone and full of statistics. After about 45 minutes of this sort of treatment even the most fractious audience can be subdued and, with careful management, the speaker can leave time only for a vote of thanks before his departure to his next engagement — which also serves to underline the good fortune of the meeting in being granted so much time out of the life of a very busy man.

For my first encounter with the BMA I eschewed such poltroonery and tried to use it as an opportunity to begin what I hoped would be a productive dialogue with the medical profession. As a dialogue, my extended question-and-answer session with the BMA, Northern Region, was not a great success. From the floor doctor after doctor told horror tales of the deteriorating condition of the NHS which illustrated the need for the Government to spend still more money, while I riposted with statistics about the government's honourable record, homilies on the economic realities which even doctors should not try to escape and earnest re-affirmations of the Conservative Party's total and immutable commitment to the national monument that is the health service.

The last contribution from the floor came from a young Lancashire GP who angrily rejected all the encouraging statistics I had put before him and said that if I came to his surgery I would soon change my tune. Then I would see his waiting room crowded with retired people who were struggling to eke out a miserable existence on the inadequate pension, many of them threatened with hypothermia or waiting many months before they could be admitted to hospital to have their badly-needed hip operation.

I could, of course, only respond with facts and national facts, at that — which, as I was to learn in my time at the DHSS, were never an effective counter to this sort of emotional assault. I pointed out that the retirement pension now bought more than it ever had in the past, that the Conservative success in reducing inflation meant that old people's savings held their value better than before, that more and more people were now being treated in our hospitals, that the rise in hip replacement operations was particularly notable and that the increase in the number of doctors had meant that, as a national average, the number of patients on a general practitioner's list had been significantly reduced.

None of this appeared to impress my truculent questioner. I was rescued by one of the oldest members of the audience who got up to say that, whilst he did not doubt the pressures felt by his young colleague, as one who had entered general practice before the NHS had been launched he viewed the situation from a different and more optimistic perspective. In the 1940s many of the sort of people who were now lining up at the doctors' surgeries would "have taken two aspirins and gone to bed for a couple of days". They had then accepted much more readily the ills of the human condition and the frailties of old age. He did not lament the change in attitudes but believed that it was something that should not be ignored.

It is a fact that has consistently been ignored, or at least underestimated, since 1949. It has been pointed out from time to time by Health Ministers (usually after leaving office) but there has been no disposition to recognise the reality of the challenge that it poses to the fundamental principles on which the NHS is based. The citadel is too strong to attack. Thus, after his stint at the Ministry, Enoch Powell noted:

> ... there is virtually no limit to the amount of medical care an individual is capable of absorbing. The moment it was established that the cervical smear test enabled incipient or prospective cancer to be diagnosed, this check-up became a "need" of every woman between the relevant ages. But we would all benefit from having our incipient or suspected ailments detected and treated sooner ... Not only is the range of treatable conditions huge and rapidly growing, there is also a vast range of quality in the treatment of those conditions. Every general practitioner knows that he palliates with pills psychiatric or psycho- logical disorders to which a great amount of skill and care could be justifiably (in a professional sense) devoted. There is hardly a type of condition from the most trivial to the gravest which is not susceptible of alternative treatments under conditions affording a wide range of skill, care, comfort, privacy, efficiency and so on ... Finally, there is the multiplier effect of successful medical treatment. Improvement in expectation of survival results in lives that demand further medical care. The lower (medically speaking) the quality of lives preserved by advancing medical science the more intense are the demands they continue to make. In short, the appetite for medical treatment *vient en mangeant*.[2]

Yet even Enoch Powell, who many would claim to be one of the most logical thinkers of his generation and the politician least likely to shrink from the harshness of reality, was not ready to go in the direction he was signalling so clearly. In the words of his biographer, T. E. Utley, "what he did not do was to contemplate, even for a moment, any fundamental change in the (NHS)." A few years later, as the first Secretary of State of the newly-created DHSS, Richard Crossman noted the same phenomenon — and demonstrated the same unwillingness to respond to it. In 1969 he said: "The pressure of demography, the pressure of technology, the pressure of democratic equalisation will always together be suffi- cient to make the standard of social services regarded as essential to a civilised community far more expensive than that community can afford. It is a complete delusion to believe that if we had no further balance of payments difficulties social service Ministers would be able to relax and assume that a kindly Chancellor will let each one of them have all the money he wants to expand his service. The trouble is that there is no foreseeable limit of the social services which the nation can reasonably require except the limit that the Government imposes."[3]

Two decades after Powell and Crossman were writing, the trends and pressures they noted are even stronger. The advance of medical science, increasingly an international phenomenon rapidly communicated to the general public, has continued at a geometric rate, thus fuelling a widespread belief that there is virtually no sickness or infirmity that cannot be cured or at least palliated if sufficient resources are devoted to it. Many of us now seem to assume that whatever ailments afflict us, however much we abuse our bodies by smoking, alcohol, stress, bad diet or lack of exercise, if we fall ill someone will be able to cure us — and if they do not that is the result of someone else's failure properly to organise or fund health care.

Like people in most other countries, we are now living longer. Whilst our depressingly high ranking in international tables for coronary heart disease underlines that our record in preventive medicine should be much better, in general our health has continued to improve steadily. This is due not only to enhanced medical services and more effective (though often very much more expensive) drugs, but also to better housing and more sensible diets and life-styles. The result is a population that is ageing and is therefore an increasingly heavy burden on the health services.

The extent of this burden was well illustrated by figures given in a House of Commons debate in November, 1985 on NHS expenditure for 1983/4. They showed the difference in spending levels as follows:

	Over 75s	Average of all age groups	16–64 age group
Hospital and Community Health Services	£875	£185	£95
Family Practitioner Services	£135	£65	£55

The final source of constant pressure for increased spending on the NHS which, although mentioned earlier, deserves a closer look is that which comes from within the service itself. It is generated by the wide range of groups in the service sometimes motivated purely by a desire to protect and improve the NHS, sometimes only by their own sectional interest and usually by a mixture of the two in which the different strands are impossible to unravel. In recent years the Royal College of Nursing has played an increasingly prominent, and sometimes even strident, role but its political effectiveness probably still falls some way short of that developed over generations by the leaders of the medical profession. The nurses are an emotional cause enjoying strong public support which in the years since 1979 has — justifiably — won them significant increases in their real pay, a shorter working week, a bigger recruitment and an independent Pay Review Board. Despite all this, however, their pay is still low by most criteria and comparisons. The doctors have done very much better, both in the level of earnings they have achieved and in the power they have continued to exert on the NHS.

The medical profession has been successful in these endeavours not only because of the highly professional campaigning and lobbying of the British Medical Association but also because of the sorties into the public arena by very many individual doctors, usually hospital consultants. Not surprisingly, the media are delighted to run tales furnished to them by doctors of alarming deficiencies and shortcomings in the National Health Service.

Every politician who has held office in the DHSS will have his own fund of stories to illustrate the highly politicised attitudes of some members of the medical profession. One occasion which left a deep impression on me was a visit I paid to a large regional teaching hospital which, justifiably, enjoys a high reputation. When I arrived at one of the wards I was greeted, affably enough, by the eminent consultant in charge, Professor X. Hearing an Australian accent, by way of an opening conversational gambit I asked how he came to be working in Britain. He said that after leaving Australia he had spent some years at a very prestigious hospital in the United States before coming to this country about ten years previously. He then launched into a set-piece and well planned attack on the allegedly appalling state of the NHS generally and especially of the hospital and on the Government's responsibility for that situation. Not only the ward sister but also the patients had clearly been briefed to sing the same tune. Indeed, so perfect was their harmony that to a large extent the effect was lost. Undoubtedly, the consultant and the hospital could have put more resources to very good use but the little demonstration was so obviously a put-up job that its impact was weakened.

I resented the attempt to turn the visit to the ward into a political confrontation — I was quite ready to have that at the meeting scheduled for the purpose later — and our exchanges grew a little heated. In the end, I suggested that if he found conditions in Britain quite so deplorable he might like to consider returning to the greener pastures of the United States or Australia. It turned out that, bad as he believed conditions in the NHS to be, he preferred to stay here.

Another demonstration of the political potency of the medical profession and their fight for more health spending occurred when in November 1985 I spoke to a meeting of one hundred or more Conservative ladies in Virginia Water. Normally it would be difficult to imagine a more congenial audience but this time I ran into a storm. The District Health Authority controlling Frimley Park Hospital had got itself into a tight spot and was seeking to introduce a variety of temporary economies. There is no doubt that it was under some pressure — like the other three Regional Health Authorities responsible for a part of the capital, the South West Thames Region was finding it very difficult to balance the

competing needs of Inner and Outer London and the Home
Counties — but it had also brought some of the trouble on itself by
poor management and by allowing itself to be bullied by the
doctors.

The result was a great deal of local alarm — no doubt, as regularly
happens all over the country, some of it deliberately whipped up —
about the threat to hospital services. The local press was full of
stories of the possible closure of wards or even of the whole hospital
for a period. As part of their campaign some of the staff at Frimley
Park seized on the opportunity presented by my meeting with the
Conservative ladies in Virginia Water. After my speech I invited
questions as usual. They came thick and fast, all but one focusing
on the situation at the hospital, and I decided to let them run on
and take a later train back to London. It seemed better to do that
than appear to be fleeing from the gunfire. Most of the questioners
began with something like "I used to be a ward sister at Frimley
Park ..." or "I had all my children at Frimley Park ..."

The climax was reached by the final contribution from the floor
by a gentleman obviously consumed with indignation who quickly
disclosed the reason for his presence among the Conservative
women. "I am a consultant at Frimley Park Hospital. I have never
been to a public meeting before. I want you to know, Minister, that
if things go on like this Surrey will be a dangerous place in which to
fall ill."

On the assumption that the man knew he was talking nonsense
(the assumption that he did not know would be an even more
depressing reflection on the medical profession) this struck me as
a classic demonstration of the politicisation of attitudes among
many doctors which has occurred as a result of the operation of the
NHS. I subsequently fulfilled the undertaking I gave to the
meeting to visit Frimley Park and needless to say, when matters
were looked into and the dust allowed to settle none of the
scenarios with which some of the hospital staff had alarmed the
media and the public actually came to pass. The consultant
with strange views on health cover in Surrey turned out to be
renowned locally for such attitudes and I was not surprised to be

told that he was a member of the District Health Authority.

There thus exists an extraordinarily powerful amalgam of pressures operating within and on the National Health Service to increase its spending and to generate the maximum level of political difficulty. It is not surprising therefore to find that the costs of the service have always outrun the forecasts and yet have failed to satisfy public aspirations.

But we should return to 1948. By December of that year, only five months after the Appointed Day, Bevan was obliged to tell the rest of the Cabinet that the original estimate of NHS spending for 1948-49 of £176 million would turn out to be £225 million (in fact it ended up as £340 million in England and Wales). He complained that:

> The rush for spectacles, as for dental treatment, has exceeded all expectations ... Part of what has happened has been a natural first flush of the new scheme, with the feeling that everything is free now and it does not matter what is charged up to the Exchequer.[5]

For the rest of his tenure at the Ministry of Health Bevan regularly continued to exhort and warn about the excessive burden being placed on the health budget and attacked dentists and general practitioners as the chief perpetrators of the sin of over-prescribing.

The exhortations had no discernible effect and ten years later the NHS budget had risen to £740 million. Thereafter the increase gathered ever more pace — checked only in years of particularly severe economic crises — fuelled by the rapid advances in medical techniques and also by the counter-bidding of the political parties when they pledged their commitment to health spending in successive election campaigns. Every party manifesto promised not only that the resources dedicated to the NHS would be used more effectively than in the past but that there would be significant increases in the total of resources to be committed.

Once safely installed in office, each new set of Health Ministers set about trying to get spending under better control. Even Bevan, under very strong pressure from his colleagues, was forced to agree to and publicly support legislation to impose a shilling charge on each NHS prescription in 1949 and to accept the creation of a special Cabinet Committee to keep health spending under constant review. Clement Attlee decided to chair this Committee himself.

Even Prime Ministerial intervention, however, proved ineffective and the following year Bevan was obliged to respond to mounting concern in the Cabinet about the rise in NHS spending. He invited a senior civil servant, Sir Cyril Jones, to make a study of the financial workings of the service. The Jones' report spotlighted two fundamental weaknesses. One of them had long been identified — even by Bevan himself; this was the "fundamental incompatibility between central control and local autonomy." The second was a phenomenon which had hitherto been only dimly recognised but which persisted and grew as a scandalous failure of the NHS in the decades which followed — and that is the extraordinary dearth of information about the costs of the services provided. Jones pointed out that:

"The fact is that the Ministry possesses very limited information regarding the financial administration of the hospitals of the country on the basis of which the estimates are framed; has no costing yardsticks at its disposal by which to judge the relative efficiency or extravagance of administration of various hospitals, and hence no alternative but either to accept the estimates wholesale as submitted without amendment or to apply overall cuts to the total budgets in a more or less indiscriminate manner."[5]

Sadly, Jones' recommendations for improvement were largely ignored and it is only in recent years that the NHS, in the teeth of strong resistance from much of the medical profession, has made any real progress in establishing an adequate system of costing. There is still a surprisingly long way to go to achieve a level of cost information which would be considered acceptable in most other spheres of life.

The Labour Government's next attempt to keep the health budget within acceptable bounds resulted in the famous resignation of Bevan himself. He had acquiesced in the announcement about prescription charges in 1949 with extreme reluctance and had managed subsequently to fend off pressure from his Treasury colleagues for their imposition, maintaining that — quite apart from his strong objection on grounds of principle — they were impractical. By early 1951 the Labour Party's mood had changed greatly from the heady, Utopian fervour of its post-war victory. In the election of February 1950 Labour's majority had been cut from 152 to 6 and the new Government was on the defensive, seeking to grapple with the harsh economic realities. It was a very different climate from the one in which the NHS was born. Following the death of Stafford Cripps, Hugh Gaitskell — the "dessicated calculating machine" in Bevan's phrase — was now at the Treasury and determined to exert financial discipline. After a bitter White-hall battle, the new Chancellor announced in his Budget of April 1951 that charges would be introduced for spectacles and dentures supplied on the NHS.

Several of Bevan's colleagues urged him not to rock what was then a very unstable political boat but when the Cabinet made clear that it would go ahead with legislation to implement the charges, Bevan resigned. In his resignation speech he was scathing about Gaitskell's Budget — "it united the City, satisfied the Opposition and disunited the Labour Party — all this because we have allowed ourselves to be dragged too far behind the wheels of American diplomacy." — and, in effect, laid down his political life to defend the purity of his concept of the health service:

"The Chancellor of the Exchequer is putting a ceiling on the Health Service. With rising prices the Health Service is squeezed between the artificial figure and the rising prices. What is to be squeezed out next year? Is it the upper half? When that has been squeezed out and the same principle holds good, what do you squeeze out the year after? Prescriptions? Hospital charges? Where do you stop? I have been accused of having agreed to a charge on prescriptions. That shows the danger of compromise. Because if it is pleaded against me that I agreed to the modification of the Health Service, then what will be pleaded against my Right Hon Friends next year, and indeed what answer will they have if the vandals opposite come in? What answer? The Health Service will be like Lavinia — all the limbs cut off and eventually her tongue cut out too."[6]

The charges were imposed and Bevan went into the wilderness. Six months later the Labour Party was defeated at the polls and now it was the Conservatives turn to wrestle with the octopus of NHS spending and in 1953 the new government set up the Guillebaud Committee to "suggest means, whether by modifications in organization or otherwise, of ensuring the most effective use of such Exchequer funds as may be made available, and to advise how, in view of the burdens on the Exchequer, a rising charge upon it can be avoided while providing for the maintenance of an adequate service."

These terms of reference contrast sharply with the Utopian approach to the provision of health services which had been common to nearly all British politicians only a few years earlier. Then, in the words of the 1944 White Paper, the objective had been to create comprehensive service which would furnish everyone with what they needed in the way of "the best medical and other facilities available" and that this provision would "not depend on whether they could pay for them, or any other factor irrelevant to the real need — the real need being to bring the country's full resources to bear upon reducing ill-health and promoting good health." By 1953 the limit of political aspiration was to "make the most effective use of such Exchequer funds as may be made available."

Yet Guillebaud's findings published on 25th January 1956 were disappointing even by these limited criteria. While recognizing defects in the Service's organisation and administration, the Committee found that any charge of widespread extravagance, either in expenditure or money or use of manpower, was not borne out by the evidence. They concluded:

> We have found no opportunity for making recommendations which would either produce new sources of income or reduce in a substantial degree the annual cost of the Service.
>
> In some instances, and particularly with regard to the level of hospital capital expenditure, we have found it necessary, in the interests of future efficiency, to make recommendations which will tend to increase the cost.

Consequently when, in the month following the publication of the Guillebaud Report, the Chancellor was obliged by the economic situation to announce cuts in the Government's capital spending programme, capital expenditure on hospitals was shielded from the axe. Thus another attempt to check the expansion of NHS costs ran into the sand. The hospital building programme which subsequently gathered pace in fact actually intensified the financial pressures on the NHS as the running costs of many of the hospitals built in the 1960s and '70s turned out to be much higher than those they replaced.

Meanwhile throughout the 1950s, successive Conservative Health Ministers tried what Rudolf Klein characterises as "policy-making through exhortation. Circulars poured out of the Ministry at an average of about 120 a year ..."[7] Given, however, the very high degree of operational autonomy which had been retained (or gained) by not only the medical but also the other professions in the service, the impact of the Ministerial exhortations fell a long way short of what was hoped for. The only effective means of control available at the centre was to ration the total budgets granted to health authorities. One effect of this was to perpetuate the regional disparities of health spending and standards of service which Bevan had seen as one of the main arguments against a local government based health service and which eventually led to the attempt at a better distribution under the programme of the Resource Allocation Working Party (RAWP).

From the beginning the NHS drugs bill grew at a worrying rate so that by 1958 the cost of drugs supplied by pharmacists and general practitioners (that is, excluding those prescribed in hospitals) accounted for 10% of the total budget. In an effort to control costs, the Ministry negotiated the first of a series of agreements with the pharmaceutical companies which sought to curb prices.

In the same year, in another effort to meet the rise in health spending, the Government increased the weekly NHS contributions paid by employees and employers — a move which, predictably enough, was fiercely attacked by the Labour Opposition. Dr. Edith Summerskill condemned it as a "panic measure" which would "place an additional burden on the poorest in the country." Even on the basis of the higher rates, the proportion of NHS expenditure covered by the total of contributions from employees and employers through NHS payments never reached higher than 17.2% (in 1962-63), a much smaller proportion than had been assumed when the service was launched. The proportion of the NHS budget covered by NHS contributions, which was 9.8% in the first year of operation, reduced fairly steadily after 1963, standing at 8.2% in 1980-81. It rose thereafter and represented 13.2% of the NHS funding announced for 1987-88.

Fresh attempts to ease the financial pressures of the NHS continued at not much more than yearly intervals. In 1959 the Ministry set up an Advisory Committee for Management Efficiency and the resources put into "hospital efficiency studies" grew sharply. Responding to the Plowden Report in 1961, the Government set up the Public Expenditure Survey Committee (PESC) system to control its own spending and in the health field one of its objectives was to seek "improvements in the method of making allocations of funds between the Regional Hospital Boards." In the wake of PESC came the variety of techniques designed to ensure that the tax-payers money would be used more effectively: such as cost-benefit analysis, Planning, Programming and Budgetting (PPB) and Programme Analysis Review (PAR). Whatever they may have achieved elsewhere in the public sector their impact on constraining the growth of NHS spending was negligible.

The exhortations to economise continued throughout the 1960s and '70s but frequently foundered on the rock of clinical autonomy. Unlike the United States, for example, in the NHS there was no serious attempt to control or even to investigate clinical procedures or performance. In this regard doctors in British hospitals, who had and continue to have grounds for complaint that they do not rate highly in the international league table of salaries for their profession, were more highly favoured than their colleagues in other countries. For example when, in 1974, the then Deputy Chief Medical Officer of the Ministry of Health pointed out that over £2 million a year could be saved if only lengths of stay for patients with appendicitis could be reduced to the same level as that already prevailing in the United States he was also at pains to stress that "there can be no question of telling surgeons how long their patients should be in hospital."[8]

Nearly fifteen years on, the same situation obtains, with extraordinary disparities between different consultants in the length of time they retain their patients in hospital, even, as an example, for routine cases of childbirth. It is one of the many signs that, despite all their complaints about managerial meddling and pennypinching, the doctors have for many years continued to reign supreme in the NHS to an extent unimagined by their colleagues in other countries. One of the effects of the most recent pressures on the service is that, at last, this particular iceberg has begun to melt. There is a growing sensitivity about the issue among some surgeons, who are now inclined to explain that they would give it more attention if only the relevant data were available; they are not because the hospital could not afford to buy the computer that would have been needed; the choice had to be made between a computer for some mere statistical exercise and a new piece of theatre or laboratory equipment ... etc ... etc ...

In 1976 the Labour Government was obliged to embark on yet another, and even more serious, effort to bring health spending under control when the state of the national economy forced it to turn to the International Monetary Fund for a rescue operation. As a result the hospital building programme was cut by a third and in three years out of four the pay rises awarded to nurses and other health service staff fell below the rise in the cost of living. The strikes of health workers during the notorious "winter of discontent" of 1978/9 were a major factor in Labour's defeat in May 1979.

During that election campaign all the political parties, as usual, promised that they would spend more on the NHS. That is a pledge which the Conservative Government handsomely honoured, with a real increase in spending over inflation of more than 30% in nine years — a particularly notable achievement when many other politically-sensitive spending programmes were being squeezed. At the same time they recognised the problems and hoped that these could be resolved by improved management techniques and a more efficient use of the steadily increasing volume of resources. The evidence of the 1987 election campaign, when the NHS was easily the most vulnerable Achilles heel of the Conservatives, demonstrated the futility of that hope.

The Conservatives sought improvements by a major structural reorganisation, eliminating the Area Health Authorities and by inviting Mr (later Sir) Roy Griffiths to make a critical examination of health service administration. Griffiths was the Chief Executive of the highly successful retail chain Sainsburys and it was hoped that he would be able to make proposals which would inject business efficiency and techniques into the NHS. His recommendations led to the introduction of the concept of "general management" into the service at all levels from the hospital Unit up to the NHS Supervisory Board, chaired by the Secretary of State. Every Region and District Health Authority was instructed to set in hand programmes of "cost improvement" which would "release cash" for necessary enhancement of the services provided. Authorities were cajoled into inviting outside contractors to tender for the supply of the ancillary services in hospitals — catering, cleaning and laundry. A harder look was taken at the property owned by the NHS so that where real estate was not needed it was to be sold and the proceeds used for services to patients.

All these were necessary and praiseworthy initiatives, but, conflicting as they did with a variety of vested interests, it was inevitable that they were controversial and caused political difficulties for the Government. What the DHSS considered to be a cost-improvement, for example, could be attacked by its critics as a "cut". The House of Commons All-Party Public Accounts Committee pursued this line in its 1986 Report: "we cannot emphasise strongly enough that cost improvement programmes should not include savings from cuts in services and we trust the measures being used by the DHSS ... will provide a greater degree of assurance as to the validity of cost improvements put forward by Regions."[9]

I shall explore later the question of whether these are areas which offer scope for further development and the possibility of making a significant contribution to the solutions of the problems of the NHS. For the purpose of this brief review of attempts to control health spending over forty years, it is sufficient to record here that the savings that all these efforts achieved in the first five years were quite incommensurate with the political damage caused. In 1984/5, for example, cost improvement programmes produced a "cash release" of £105 million — which appears a considerable sum until it is set against the expenditure of some £10,000 million on hospital and community health services during that year.

Thus, from the first year of its operation, every government has made determined attempts to keep the NHS budget under control. All these efforts, only a selection of which have been mentioned above, have failed when judged by the rise in health spending — which has regularly been higher under Conservative than under Labour administrations — so that it went from £433 million in calendar year 1949 to £19,624 million in the financial year 1986/7. Using the standard GDP deflator to allow for the effects of inflation, this represents *a real increase of no less than 280%*.

The deepest irony is that this huge growth has almost certainly been outmatched by the rise in public concern about the state of the NHS over the period. Whilst the evidence of opinion polls suggests that the level of satisfaction with the service of those who have recently been patients remains high, it is also clear that the electorate increasingly perceives the service as being subjected to a remorselessly tightening budget squeeze.

Among those with a professional concern in the health field there is a widely-held view that there must be an annual growth of at least 2% and indeed this figure was accepted by the Conservative Government. For example, responding to a Report prepared by the Centre for Health Economics at the University of York for the Institute of Health Service Management, the British Medical Association and the Royal College of Nursing in December 1986, my colleague, Barney Hayhoe, then Minister of Health, wrote:

"I agree that, as the Report suggested, health authority services need at present to grow by about 2% a year in order to meet the pressures they face. One per cent is needed to keep pace with the increasing number of very elderly people (although this pressure is now at a peak and will decline into the 1990s); medical advance takes an additional 0.5% and a further 0.5% is needed to make progress towards meeting the Government's policy objectives (for example to improve renal services and develop community care)." He went on, however, to "emphasise that it is services and not expenditure that need to grow by 2%. Services are developed both by increased cash allocations and by greater efficiency in the use of resources."

This caveat is not, of course, accepted by political parties when they are in opposition nor by the health service professionals. Thus in a joint memorandum sent to the Chancellor of the Exchequer in 1986 the BMA, RCN and the Institute of Health Service Management argued for an interpretation which would provide "additional funding of the order of 2% per annum *excluding* provision for pay and price inflation and capital expenditure."

The fact is that since 1949 government spending on the NHS, after allowing for price inflation, has increased at an annual *average rate of 3.67%* yet the unmet demand and political dissatisfaction have grown to levels which are so serious that it is now clear that fundamental changes are inescapable.

Bevan's "cascade of medicine" has become a massively rising cascade of medical advance and higher demand which is engulfing the service for which he was proud to claim so much responsibility. It is a phenomenon which is by no means unique to Britain; in every country the demand for better health care rises sharply as prosperity increases. But it is a problem which in this country, because of the characteristics of the NHS, is uniquely difficult to solve.

5
Changing the Structure

The funding problem of the National Health Service, virtually ignored in the decades of debate which preceded its launch, has proved resistant to forty years of unremitting effort at its solution. Indeed, the problem has got much worse and, unless fundamental changes are made, there is no doubt it will continue to do so.

The same is true of a problem which *was* foreseen and debated exhaustively before the Appointed Day: the difficulty of finding a structure which can be controlled and funded centrally but which also responds to local, professional and individual requirements and is able to deliver all aspects of health care in a satisfactory and coordinated manner. Despite the plethora of studies and reports and two major reorganisations since 1948, no-one could seriously claim that the present arrangements have come near to resolving the dilemma.

As we have seen in earlier chapters, this was an issue of fierce debate between the members of the post-war Labour Cabinet. Herbert Morrison complained that Bevan's scheme would result in bureaucratic over-centralisation. Bevan pinned his faith on selecting the right people to serve on the Regional Boards and District Committees but also hoped that the future would bring "development in the field of government" which would provide solutions to the problems Morrison had identified.

It was always an unrealistic hope and another example of Bevan's natural tendency to deal with the world as he would have liked it to be rather than the world as it is. Such a tendency is not in the least surprising in a romantic, between-the-wars socialist — and (if an Englishman may risk a racist observation) a Welshman to boot. What is surprising is that virtually the whole of the rest of the nation seems to have shared the same unjustified optimism for so many decades. It is one more demonstration of the uncanny power of the mystique of the NHS to paralyse normal political thought in Britain.

When it was launched in 1948 the National Health Service was created as a tripartite structure — the hospitals, family practitioners and the various community services. Then, as ever since, the hospitals attracted most public attention and absorbed most of health service spending — currently it accounts for about two-thirds of the total. The Minister of Health became responsible for the hospitals, all of them now brought into the "nationalised" system, administering them through fourteen Regional Hospital Boards. The teaching hospitals were kept outside this arrangement and each had its own Board of Governors reporting directly to the Minister. The non-teaching hospitals were run on a day-to-day basis by Hospital Management Committees appointed by the RHBs.

The functions of the Regional Boards were not clearly laid down either in the NHS Act or any related legislation: they tended to emerge, helped by various statutory instruments and Ministry memoranda. Their essential role was to plan and develop the hospital and specialist services within the region and within the budgetary limits set by the Minister. They exercised quite a tight control over the Hospital Management Committees, especially over staffing matters.

The Regional Boards acquired one responsibility which has developed into an issue of some importance and contention: they became the direct employer of all the consultants and specialists working in the hospitals in the region. The aim of this arrangement was to achieve the most effective and flexible use of skilled medical manpower and ensure that it was properly deployed throughout the region rather than concentrated in certain favoured hospitals.

Increasingly, and particularly in recent years, this has come to be regarded by the doctors as one of the major bulwarks defending their professional autonomy and therefore fiercely defended as such. In any clash between their clinical freedom and the efforts of general managers at hospital or district level to secure the most economic use of resources, consultants regularly take advantage of the fact that their contracts are still with the Regional Authority.

Members of the Regional Hospital Boards were appointed by the Minister of Health after consultation with the relevant universities, medical organisations, local authorities and any other agency he considered appropriate. Bevan seemed to make a serious effort to ensure that the membership of each Board, which numbered between twenty and thirty, achieved a reasonable cross-section of society — with the occasional misfits virtually inevitable in such cases. As no fees were paid, however, the great majority of members tended to come from particular groups: the retired, professional people or nominees of organisations.

An analysis of those appointed to the first Regional Boards showed that 29% were doctors and dentists — a significant figure — 15% were women and 85% had previous experience with hospitals in some capacity or other.[1]

The Boards were served by a staff of salaried permanent officials, including medical advisers. As is normally the case with such arrangements, the officials and the Chairman have usually been able to carry the rest of the Members along with them.

Unlike the hospital sector, the creation of the NHS brought relatively few changes to the family practitioner service. The objective was to change as little as possible the doctor-patient relationship which had existed under the old system of private medical practice. The family doctor was to act as the "gatekeeper" controlling patient access to the hospitals. Another significant difference between the family practitioner and the hospital services was that, from the beginning of the NHS, it was always the latter which was subjected to direct financial constraints. When, in 1976, the Treasury introduced formal "cash limits" to some of its spending programmes it fought very hard, and successfully, to get the hospital services included. The family practitioner service has survived without a cash limit. This is why the hospitals and those who work in them have always had to fight for their funds — and have therefore always been at the centre of nearly every political battle.

The general practitioners were "independent contractors" but were administered through Executive Councils, 138 of which were created in England and Wales. They covered the same areas as the counties and county boroughs but were independent of them — the doctors having consistently demonstrated their hostility to the concept of municipal control. Each Executive Council had twenty-five members but the Minister of Health had the right to appoint only five. Of the remainder, eight were appointed by the local authority, seven by the local doctors, three by the dentists and two by the pharmacists. They were served by a permanent staff.

One important role of the Executive Councils was to rationalise and improve the distribution of general practitioners, something badly needed in many parts of the country in 1948.

The third element of the original NHS structure was the community services delivered by the local authorities. These included the maternity and child welfare services, health visitors, home helps and ambulances.

Doubts about Bevan's failure to create a more unified health service had been expressed by many people since at least 1946. These concerns increased once the service came into operation and prompted a virtually non-stop stream of reports and studies in the decades that followed.

Perhaps the first of significance was that produced by Sir John Maude, a member of the Guillebaud Committee set up in 1953 (see Chapter 4, page 58). The majority of the Committee, although acknowledging that there were weaknesses, did not consider that structural changes in the service were necessary at that time. Maude, however, underlines the problems caused within the NHS by the existence of three separate bodies which were funded differently and had no organic connection with each other. He believed that there was wasteful overlapping between the hospitals and the general practitioners and that the predominance of the hospital sector denied the family practitioner and community services the attention they deserved. Maude believed that responsibility for the provision of all health services should be passed to the local authorities *if* — a very difficult if, as future efforts at reform were to show — satisfactory funding arrangements could be devised.. Other countries have gone down the route of organising and funding their health services on a local or regional basis but a successful formula to resolve the dilemma between the national allocation of resources and the satisfaction of local needs has continued to elude us in Britain.

In the years after Guillebaud there came a steady stream of reports and initiatives aimed at remedying the structural and other deficiencies identified in the NHS. In 1959 the Earl of Cranbrook's Committee criticised the lack of integration between the maternity services provided by the hospitals and by local authorities. The Mental Health Act of the same year changed significantly the legislation on mental illness, reducing the grounds for compulsory admission to and detention in mental hospitals. Coinciding with the introduction of a number of new drugs and more effective treatment of psychiatric problems, this began the move for mental hospitals to discharge an increasing number of their patients back into the community. This process was still gathering momentum over a quarter of a century later, with constant wrangling between the NHS and local authorities over the funding and organisation of "care in the community". This is yet another area where a new approach is badly needed.

In 1962 a group set up by the medical profession, independently of the Ministry of Health, under the chairmanship of Sir A. Porritt, proposed that the delivery of health services should be unified under Area Health Boards. The following year, however, a report commissioned by the Ministry from a committee led by Dr Annis Gillie rejected unification in favour of a more dominant role for general practitioners. It argued that the family doctor was best placed to co-ordinate the hospital and community services needed by their patients.

Other reports focused on the problems within hospitals. By 1963 growing concern about the shortage of trained nurses and the apparent decline in the status of the profession led the Government to set up the Salmon Committee. Reporting three years later, Salmon suggested that the titles "matron" and "sister" were anachronistic and inappropriate — particularly as men were increasingly entering the profession — and made proposals which aimed to fit the role of nursing more effectively into the management system of modern hospitals. Salmon recommended a new hierarchy of Chief, Principal and Senior Nursing Officers who would take their due place in the managerial pecking order. The recommendations were adopted by the Government — but the nostalgia for "matron" and all she stood for still lingers in many hearts.

Recognition of the need to use hospital resources more effectively led to the production of a series of studies known, because of the design printed on their covers, as the "Cogwheel" Reports, the first appearing in 1967. The essence of their proposals was to increase the level of communication and quality of information available to all the professionals working in hospitals in order to improve the control of expenditure. It was argued, in Rudolf Klein's words, that "if all the consultants became aware of the effects of their individual decisions on the total use of resources ... they would themselves have an incentive to apply pressure on colleagues who used their beds wastefully: it would make it clear that one consultant's extravagance was another consultant's loss. Consultants would view beds no longer as their private property but as a common resource." With truly British under-statement, Klein concludes: "It is not clear how successful this strategy was."[2] Over twenty years later the new-style general managers were still complaining that these admirable principles were still too often more honoured in the breach than the observance. Some consultants still tended to consider that they "owned" patients and were unwilling to lose them. They also accepted direct referrals from general practitioners without the knowledge of the District Health Authorities, thus making for difficulties of control.

A major initiative to examine the structure of the NHS was announced in the House of Commons in November 1967 by Kenneth Robinson, then Minister of Health in the Labour Government. This resulted, eight months later, in the publication of *The Administrative Structure of Medical and Related Services in England and Wales*, which subsequently became known as the *First Green Paper*. This document resurrected yet again the proposal that all the health services provided in a locality should be unified under a new body to be called an Area Board, some forty to fifty such Boards to be established in England and Wales, serving populations of between 750,000 and three million.

Two other related reports appeared in the same period. The Seebohm Committee recommended that all personal social services should be unified into departments under the control of local authorities. The Royal Commission on Local Government in England, under the chairmanship of Lord Redcliffe-Maud, recommended the creation of new unitary authorities grouped into eight provinces each with its own provincial council. It believed that unitary authorities would be well fitted to take over the responsibilities for co-ordinating health services on the lines set out in the First Green Paper and to integrate personal social services as advocated by Seebohm. The Commission recognised that the funding of the health services would represent a massive burden but hoped that a solution could be found. None ever was and of these three sets of recommendations only Seebohm was adopted, being implemented in the Local Authority (Social Services) Act 1970.

It was next the turn of Richard Crossman to wrestle with the NHS leviathan when he succeeded Kenneth Robinson to become the first Secretary of State for Social Services in the new Department of Health and Social Security in 1968. He published *The Future Structure of the National Health Service*, known as the *Second Green Paper*, in February 1970. Crossman rejected much of the First Green Paper and Redcliffe-Maud and stuck far more closely to the *status quo*. He accepted the need for new health authorities with boundaries "co-terminous" with those of local government; they were, however, to be independent of local authorities, responsible to and funded by the DHSS through the Regional Health Councils. Public health and personal social services would continue to be the responsibility of the local authorities.

The general election of June 1970 produced a Conservative Government and Sir Keith Joseph took over at the DHSS. He carried on with the attempt to improve the efficiency of the NHS which finally emerged as the National Health Service Reorganisation Act 1973. Joseph's proposals further diluted the recommendations of the Second Green Paper but their main thrust towards a greater degree of unification of services was supported by both major parties as there was a widespread recognition of the need for improvement. The structure which emerged included strong Regional Health Authorities, with Area Health Authorities and District Management Teams operating below them. Hospitals, health centres and community nursing services were grouped under the new authorities, general practitioners continued to be administered and financed separately through Family Practitioner Committees and the local authority retained responsibility for personal social services. A new agency for the consumer's voice was introduced with the creation of Community Health Councils, outside the chain of authority. Labour objected to the complexity of the new structure, their spokesman the late John Silkin advising the Government "if you have tiers, prepare to shed them now." — advice ignored when Labour returned to office but followed by a Conservative Government ten years later.

The reorganisation of the NHS, which took effect in 1974, quickly ran into trouble. It soon became clear that the arrangements for decision making were too cumbersome and remote and were subject to excessive consultation. Moreover, the structural complexity led to greater bureaucracy. The number of administrative and clerical staff rose from 87,000 in 1973 to 113,000 in 1976.

It was during these years that the new Labour Government, which took office in 1974, became locked into a bitter political battle with the medical profession. The immediate cause of the dispute was over the question of private beds in NHS hospitals but the issues at stake went very much wider. In October, 1974 the Presidents of the Royal Colleges and the Deans of the medical faculties issued a statement which included the following: "The ills within the NHS are serious and by threatening standards threaten the health and well-being of the community. There is a real danger of standards deteriorating to a point from which recovery will be impossible within a foreseeable term."[3]

This was very similar to the protest issued by the Presidents of the Royal Colleges in December, 1987 (Chapter 1, page 11) and which was hailed by Labour politicians and others as "unprecedented". There is nothing new about the pressures on the NHS or the fears of "deteriorating standards". What is now new, after forty years, is a dawning realisation that our predecessors probably made some fundamental errors in believing that the NHS structure was likely to be the best means of delivering comprehensive health care.

The Labour Government found itself in difficulty not only with the doctors but also with NHS workers in the lower grades, among whom was developing a growing spirit of militancy. In response to these concerns Barbara Castle, then Secretary of State for Social Services, set up yet another inquiry into the NHS in May 1976. She invited Sir Alec Merrison, Vice Chancellor of Bristol University, to chair a Royal Commission with the following terms of reference: "To consider in the interests both of the patients and of those who work in the National Health Service, the best use and management of the financial and manpower resources of the National Health Service."

The Merrison Commission, which comprised 16 members and cost nearly £1 million, took three years over its deliberations. When it reported in July 1979 it concluded "we need not be ashamed of our health service and that there are many aspects of it of which we can be justly proud." Nevertheless it recorded many penetrating criticisms — shortage of funds, worsening industrial relations, longer hospital waiting lists, the absence of criteria by which to judge efficiency and the "debilitating" effects of the 1974 reorganisation. The Report noted that whilst Britain was spending less on health than most other advanced countries, in relation both to its population and to its national income, the proportion of our gross domestic product devoted to it continued to rise — from 5.3% in 1974 to 5.6% in 1977 — and in terms of medical and nursing staff employed we were doing better than the differences in expenditure would lead one to expect, thanks to lower costs and salaries in the NHS. Even so, Britain was in 1974 performing "relatively poorly" in terms of three indicators of health — life expectancy and perinatal and maternal mortality — although it was recognised that no single mortality statistic or group of statistics can summarise the health of a nation.

The Commission reported that they had "received several proposals for changing arrangements for financing the NHS" in order to supplement or replace the Exchequer spending, which by 1978/9 comprised 88% from general taxation, 9.5% from National Insurance contributions and 2.5% from charges. However, despite the disturbing pressures on NHS resources and the shortcomings they discovered, like all other official investigators into the health service before or since — so far — Sir Alec Merrison and his colleagues shied away from any significant new ideas about funding.

They did resurrect an old idea for organisational change — that the Regional Health Authorities should become virtually autonomous and "accountable to Parliament for matters within their competence." But this proposal foundered on the rock that had sunk similar suggestions in the past. The Commission recognised that the task of "apportioning revenue and capital funds between RHAs ... (would) clearly have to be undertaken centrally" but they thought "these problems could be overcome." The fact is that, as much earlier experience had demonstrated, they could not and the Commission's proposals would have created a structure which would have been unacceptable either to Members of Parliament, who understandably wish to hold Ministers to account for the health care of their constituents, nor to the Government of the day, which would be unlikely to tolerate RHAs operating as independent fiefdoms. It was another example of the woolly thinking that has plagued the provision of adequate health services in this country for so many years.

The Commission endorsed the widely held view that one of the mistakes of the 1974 reorganisation had been to create one tier of administration too many and recommended that there should be only one level of authority beneath the region. This was the principal recommendation picked up by the new Conservative Government which had taken office two months before the Commission reported.

The Conservatives issued a consultative document, *Patients First*, in December 1979. It was a slender document in contrast to the volumes published by the Royal Commission and concentrated on management issues; they were understandably nervous about launching the NHS into yet another major upheaval. The essence of Patrick Jenkin's proposals was to abolish the Area Health Authorities and, in the words of my predecessor but one, Sir George Young, "to have decisions taken as near to the point of delivery of the service as possible." There was a new emphasis on localism and a reaction against the technological planning and expertise concentrated in giant District General Hospitals which had dominated NHS thinking in the 1960s.

The new approach involved the abandonment of the principle of "coterminosity". On the face of it the idea that health authorities should have common boundaries with county councils (or in metropolitan counties, with district councils) seemed sensible. But in many cases these boundaries did not reflect arrangements for medical care which had long been established or the natural catchment areas of District General Hospitals.

The proposals in *Patients First* were passed into legislation and put into effect from 1982. The 90 Area Health Authorities were replaced by 192 DHAs, working through 14 RHAs, who emerged from the reorganisation with a somewhat more powerful role. A quarter of the membership of DHAs was reserved for local councillors, a reduction from the minimum of one third representation on AHAs which Labour had introduced in 1975. Labour's other proposal to include at least two further members in each AHA "drawn from amongst those working in the NHS" had run into the sand because of disagreements among the trade unions and between the unions and the professional organisations. Under the new arrangements one member of each DHA was to be appointed on the recommendation of the trade unions, together with a consultant, a general practitioner and a nurse.

The abandonment of coterminosity was one move away from the goal of the unification of the delivery of health and related services which had frequently been accepted but never achieved since at least 1948. Another was the decision taken by the Conservatives in their 1982 reorganisation to confirm the Family Practitioner Committees as free-floating bodies, with their boundaries and finances entirely independent of the DHA. The Royal Commission, reflecting the perceived need to integrate general practice more closely with the hospital and other health services, had recommended the abolition of the FPCs. The Government backed away, however, recognising that the proposal would lead to a serious confrontation with the general practitioners. It was another example of the power of the medical profession to hold up reform of the NHS.

The possibility of a serious examination of ways to reform opened up in September 1982 but it was quickly and unceremoniously stifled. Like Enoch Powell and others before her, Margaret Thatcher found the prospect too daunting. It occurred as the Cabinet was embarking on its annual round of battles to control the rise in public spending. The Central Policy Review Staff — the Think Tank — had produced a paper outlining a set of radical policy options in the areas of health, social security, education and defence which would have led to cuts in public spending. According to *The Economist*, to which the contents of the paper were leaked, the report was circulated to all members of the Cabinet with the endorsement of the Chancellor of the Exchequer, Sir Geoffrey Howe, and the Chief Secretary, Leon Brittan, who recommended a six-month study of the proposals. On health, the paper proposed that the NHS should be replaced by a system of insurance — which, it was estimated, could save £3-4 billion a year from a budget, in 1982-83, of £10 billion.

The paper immediately created a storm within the Cabinet and because of this it was not discussed, as had been intended, at the meeting on 9th September. The storm became very much greater when its contents were leaked and Ministerial differences came out into the open. The Government's difficulties were even greater because the episode occurred when it was locked into a fierce pay dispute with NHS staff.

The Secretary of State for Social Services, Norman Fowler, hastily leaped into the battle and pledged the Government's unshakeable commitment to the National Health Service. No. 10 let it be known that, contrary to other accounts, discussion of the paper on 9th September had been shelved at the Prime Minister's instigation. She was opposed to the recommendations. The NHS was "safe in our hands". Howe and Brittan made speeches in which they continued to insist that radical options had to be considered. But they had lost the battle; and soon afterwards Margaret Thatcher abolished the Think Tank.

The Prime Minister's rapid disavowal was not enough to stop the other political parties trying to make capital out of the affair, particularly as it broke at the time of the party conference season. At the Liberal conference in Bournemouth, for example, Cyril Smith warned the Government to keep its hands off the "people's NHS" and told a harrowing tale about when his mother had to buy a threepenny pair of spectacles from Woolworths. The battle rumbled on after Parliament resumed so that by December Mrs Thatcher was rejecting a request by the Commons Education and Science Committee to see the paper, writing to its Chairman, Christopher Price, that: "There is no such report ... The CPRS prepared a confidential analysis for ministers, outlining a number of possible ways of limiting the growth of public spending in the longer term, so that we could decide whether to commission further work on any of them. As I explained to the House of November 11 that paper was not discussed and no further work is being done on it." R.I.P.!

However, as spending and public criticism of the service both continued to escalate, the Conservatives recognised that something more needed to be done. Thus, only months after the 1982 changes began to be implemented, they set in hand yet another inquiry. This was the study by a team led by Roy Griffiths, discussed briefly in the previous chapter (page 64). The consensus management practised by the District Management Teams had meant that no one member was clearly identified as having responsibility for taking action. Not surprisingly, the result was a great deal of procrastination — much of it, according to many accusations, caused by doctors. When he reported in October 1983 Griffiths identified this weakness as the principal cause for the lack of drive he found in the NHS and therefore proposed the appointment of General Managers at Unit, District and Regional level with clearly defined roles. He also recommended the creation of a Health Service Management Board, with a Chairman, recruited from outside the NHS and the civil service, who would be vested with executive authority over the NHS derived from the Secretary of State. The Management Board was to be accountable to the Health Service Supervisory Board, chaired by the Secretary of State and comprising his junior Ministers, Permanent Secretary, the Chief Medical and Nursing Officers of the DHSS and the Chairman of the Management Board.

I believe that since 1983 there has been an improvement in the quality of management and decision-taking in the NHS and that resources are now better used. However, by none of the criteria that matter, can the Griffiths proposals be said to have come near to solving the real problems of the service; nor do they look like doing so.

There was great difficulty in recruiting the sort of high-flying managers implicit in the Griffiths concept. Such paragons can seldom be attracted by NHS salaries (even though in 1987 they were around £30,000 p.a. for the higher levels, with generous incentive bonus arrangements) or persuaded to accept the vulnerable nature of a job which is exposed to pressures from higher authority, politicians, patients, professionals within the service and the media and for which, by its nature, it is extremely difficult to construct satisfactory performance criteria. Talented people can find easier ways to make a living. As a result the great majority of the management posts were taken up by the old hospital administrators and secretaries — in my experience, a maligned body of men and women, who have been able to produce much better results when relieved of the bonds of consensus management.

The Griffiths formula, however, is inherently flawed. It has not and, I believe, cannot create a satisfactory relationship between the general manager and the chairman at the various levels. An even greater problem developed over the post of the Chairman of the Management Board and its first incumbent, Victor Paige, resigned after struggling with the job for about eighteen months. Try as he might, he could not find a role which produced a satisfactory relationship with the RHA general managers and their chairmen, the Permanent Secretary and the other senior officials of the DHSS and with the Secretary of State, the other Health Ministers and Parliament. Since Paige's resignation another reshuffle of responsibilities at the top of the NHS pyramid has been attempted but I see no prospect that the fundamental dilemmas can be resolved.

The issue over which Herbert Morrison and Aneurin Bevan battled in the Labour Cabinet of 1946 has continued to haunt the NHS ever since: how to reconcile the needs of a nationally-funded organisation with a service which is essentially local and directed towards the individual, a problem made vastly more difficult by the unique extent to which in Britain it has become politicised. As a Health Minister, one of my tasks was to conduct annual review meetings with RHA chairmen and their general managers and other colleagues. They were exercises in cajolery rather than management. To a considerable extent, once the principal budget allocation is made, the rest is up to the Region to make of it what they will. The Department aspires to set "priorities" but, inevitably, they become so numerous that they cannot all be fulfilled and the process loses its point. One Regional General Manager has totalled up no less than 46 policies and initiatives to which the DHSS has requested him to give priority. 46 priorities means no priorities.

Despite all the efforts to evolve a satisfactory set of relationships and responsibilities between the DHSS, the Regions and the Districts, it remains the case that when things go wrong in Upper

Puddlecombe general hospital, little or nothing is heard from the Chairmen or general managers along the line whose decisions are likely to have caused the problem. Parliament and the media want to hear from the Ministers who, in constitutional terms, carry the responsibility. It is a classic example of how not to organise public affairs.

Forty years of debate, enquiries, reports and changes have only brought us to the present highly unsatisfactory situation. Surely it must now be recognised that as it was constituted in 1948, the National Health Service is a failure in terms of its structure and organisation, its funding and — most importantly — in the quality of the care it delivers to the British people. Forty years of tinkering have not produced the answers we need and there is no prospect that they can ever be found without new thinking and courageous political leadership.

6

Can We Make the Straitjacket More Comfortable?

To turn away from the harshness of reality and the need to take painful decisions is an entirely normal tendency. It is one to which we in Britain are, perhaps, even more prone than most other people — despite the beneficial changes in attitudes and in society which have occurred since 1979. It is therefore not surprising, given the general perception of the continuing power of the NHS myth, that British politicians resolutely ignore the obvious message of the failure of forty years of tinkering with Bevan's creation.

All Health Ministers quickly come to understand that it is a straitjacket which prevents the development of health services which would truly match up to modern aspirations and to the possibilities of contemporary medicine. Their consciousness of the political "realities", however, allows them to be persuaded that it is a straitjacket they can live in at least long enough to get their Government safely past the next general election and themselves happily into the next Ministerial post.

Nearly all the advice they are given pushes them in the same direction. Their Party colleagues are quick to remind them of the potency of the health issue — "sick baby turned away from hospital" or "our underpaid angels, the nurses" are powerfully emotive themes which the media and opposition politicians are very happy to exploit. The officials who fill their working days and the Ministerial boxes they take home in the evenings are, *ex officio*, committed to the survival and expansion of the NHS and see their principal role to be to arm their Ministers with the most effective weapons to extract more tribute out of the Treasury in their regular battles with the Chief Secretary. With diligence and luck it is possible to discover one or two officials who are prepared to consider the possibility that Mr Bevan's formula might not, after all, have been the most sensible way of delivering health care to the British people — but the open expression of such heresy, which goes against all the traditions and habits of the Department, is about as rare as was the advocacy of toleration for the Jews in Hitler's Germany.

The message that all will be well provided you can extract just a little more money from the Chancellor is also powerfully delivered to Health Ministers in their daily contacts with the NHS itself. It starts near at hand with the advice they are given by the Chief Medical Officer and the Chief Nursing Officer and their respective staffs — much more the voice of the professions directed at the Government than genuine two-way conduits — and is reinforced by every meeting with luminaries of the Royal Colleges, the BMA, the RCN and the rest and by every visit to a hospital or health centre. They also hear the same theme from the Chairmen of the Regional and District Health Authorities — and often put more effectively. The Chairmen are not usually medical professionals themselves and will have been appointed by the current batch of Ministers or their predecessors; they are therefore regarded, usually rightly, as approaching the problem with a much greater degree of detachment and objectivity. However, often under the tutelage of their general manager, they absorb the ethos and traditional attitudes of the NHS with remarkable speed and intensity and certainly see their role as improving the system rather than proposing fundamental changes. New thinking on the NHS is a very rare commodity.

The forces defending the *status quo* are therefore very strong and operate not only on Health Ministers but on the whole Government. Yet the paradox exists and deepens, as we have already seen:

more and more public resources are devoted to the NHS but public dissatisfaction with the service continues to escalate. In such a situation the natural political reaction is to complain that "the message is not getting across; that is what we need to do better." In the years after 1979, that was the cry heard increasingly in Conservative meetings up and down the country, from Tory Members of Parliament and from Ministers not directly saddled with the task of delivering the message. It is always easier to shoot the pianist than to compose a new tune, particularly one with the extraordinary characteristics of the NHS, and I write as one of the assassinated pianists.

We were fighting an unwinnable battle. Quite apart from the fundamental problem that is the essence of this book — that whilst we have a system that allows us, as a nation, to spend only about 6% of our GDP on health we shall never have a service which comes near to meeting present or future demand — we suffered grievously from the media maxim that good news is rarely news. The opening of a new multi-million pound general hospital might rate a few paragraphs in the local paper and, if we were lucky with the VIP cutting the tape, even a photograph. But there would be no coverage in the national media. Yet if a particular ward was closed — often because it needed to be because much more modern and better-sited facilities had been built to replace it — the national press would cheerfully carry dramatic pictures, often accompanied by a harrowing story from a hospital porter who would now have to travel a little further to his work.

The nadir of this type of journalism has regularly been reached by the *Daily Mirror*. For a year or two before the 1987 general election, no doubt recognising this as the most promising ground on which to attack the Conservative Government, the paper ran a ferocious campaign against the funding of the health service. *Mirror* readers were encouraged to tell of any problems they had encountered with the NHS. With such an organisation, dealing with millions of patients every year, stories of delay and disappointment are not too hard to find. The *Mirror* milked them for all they were worth — and much more. Naturally we investigated all the allegations and I sought to correct the more outrageous distortions. Such effrontery on my part inevitably incurred the wrath of the *Mirror* and so they paid me the compliment of turning their fire on to me. "You're a liar, Mr Whitney" screamed their banner headlines, after I had corrected one particularly slanted story.

Recall of this episode prompts to a brief digression on the present state of our libel laws. Needless to say, I had certainly *not* lied in correcting the *Mirror*'s tendentious story and in my innocence of our court procedures I thought I would have a cast-iron case against them. Indeed, when I mentioned the affair to a friend who is a very experienced journalist and jested that damages paid by the *Mirror* might cover my forthcoming holiday in Crete, his reaction was that "they will buy you bloody Crete." For understandable reasons, Governments shy away from legal entanglements with newspapers but I decided to pursue my battle with the *Mirror* on a personal basis, not least because I had been left to wage it alone by my Ministerial colleagues. However, I had second thoughts when I obtained advice from a leading and very sympathetic libel lawyer. Although he accepted that the facts were totally in my favour — I manifestly had not lied — he could only rate my chances of success at what he described as 85:15, the best odds he could ever forecast for any potential client in a libel case. The uncertainty (in a case where, in reality as opposed to in law, there was no uncertainty) arises from the element of chance involved in the composition of the jury. The existing system frequently produces juries which, even when presented with overwhelming evidence, cannot be guaranteed to bring in verdicts in favour of what some of their members might regard as "the establishment". Given the certainty of astronomical legal costs, the likelihood of only modest damages ("politicians must expect that sort of treatment") and the odds I had been quoted, it clearly did not make sense for me to take on the *Mirror* and Maxwell's millions. Such a situation is deeply unhealthy and is especially surprising to find in a country which prides itself on having enjoyed for so long the rule of law and the benefits of democracy.

There was a consoling footnote to my battles with the *Daily*

Mirror. One day I was paying a visit to the Moorfields Eye Hospital in central London, which does splendid work and was coping well with the problems of an extensive rebuilding programme on a very restricted site. I came to the bed of a tiny old lady who radiated such Cockney cheerfulness that she might even have appeared a cliché in a Noel Coward production. She had been afflicted with eye problems nearly all her life and had been a patient at Moorfield roughly every five years. I asked her what changes she had found and what she thought about all the talk of cuts and deterioration in the NHS. She would have none of that. Moorfield was marvellous and things were better every time she came in. I noted that she had a *Daily Mirror* on her bedside locker. I suggested she might write to give the paper her views, as they were so ready to publicise criticisms of the NHS. Her reply was revealing. "They'd never print it, luv," she said.

The 1987 election campaign and the run-up to it convinced all Conservative politicians, from Margaret Thatcher downwards, that the problems created by the NHS could not be solved simply by "better presentation". During that period we all came to know by heart the standard defence of our record in producing more resources for the service which, as a Health Minister, I had chanted like a mantra throughout the country. The response of hostile questioners — and I do not believe it is paranoia when I say that nearly all were hostile — tended to be: "we do not wish to hear how much more is being spent on the NHS, how many more patients are being treated or how many more doctors and nurses are employed. We want to know why Mr Smith must wait so long for his operation or why Upper Puddlecombe Memorial Hospital is being closed." After the general election the understanding that there was a need for something more than media management came to be widely accepted.

This led to increased emphasis being given to a point of view which had been current for years in a number of quarters, notably H.M.Treasury, that if only the NHS could be brought to use properly the vast and increasing resources devoted to it, all would be well. This line is sometimes accompanied by sorrowful recollections of halcyon days in the mythical past when the NHS was not plagued with armies of bureaucrats and "general managers" and when Matron ruled her domain with ferocious efficiency and economy.

The evidence available gives no support to the view that the problems of the NHS can be solved by a more effective use of resources. On the contrary, whilst it will always be possible to find examples of poor administration and control in a structure of the size and nature of the NHS, many indications suggest that, on the basis of international comparisons, the overhead costs of the service are not high. In relation to the money we, as a nation, spend the NHS does not represent too bad a deal. Certainly it at least provides us with a good *emergency* service.

Comparisons in this field are notoriously difficult to make. Where, for example, are the limits to be drawn in defining overhead costs? Should they include the salary of a consultant's personal assistant or a ward secretary? Which indicators should be used to give a profile of a nation's health — for example, the number of patients treated as a percentage of the population, life expectancy, infant mortality, the percentage provided with renal or other special treatments etc etc? And what is the extent to which some of these indicators are affected by factors unrelated to the quality of the health service?

Such difficulties make a definitive judgement impossible. However the consensus of many experts suggests that the NHS probably uses its resources at least as well as most health systems in the developed world. Two American observers suggest that British administrative costs probably amount to some 6% of total expenditure while putting the United States figure — of a much higher level of spending — at about 10%. Such comparisons tend to flatter the British performance as they do not include an element for the collection costs of revenue in a centrally funded system whereas they do include those costs in an insurance system; thus there is an under-estimate of our administrative costs compared with the basis used to calculate overheads in the United States.

Nevertheless, given that even after the forty years of striving that we have already discussed, costing and incentive mechanisms are rudimentary or non-existent in the NHS, it is surprising that we have done so well. Much of the explanation for this achievement, of course, lies in the relatively low pay levels — especially by international standards in terms of purchasing power — which exist in the service. One result of the situation is that while we do relatively well in the provision of what is now regarded as traditional treatment, the NHS is slow to adopt new technologies.

Governments will, rightly, continue to insist that the service maintains its efforts to hold its administrative costs in check — but the difficulties and drawbacks involved are certain to increase. Nearly every NHS insider will assert strongly that the service has already been pared to the bone and there is no more fat to be taken off. Without necessarily accepting this case, there is no doubt that future *additional* savings will only be possible, if they can be achieved at all, with even greater political damage than has been sustained so far.

Further efforts at cost-holding, let alone cost-cutting, will lead to ever fiercer media battles between the medical and nursing professions on the one hand and the NHS management on the other. It will always be a desperately unequal contest. The concerned and caring professionals, who have learned a great deal about this particular game over the years, will always vanquish the hard-faced, narrow and insensitive bureaucrats. The struggles so far have already resulted in the concept of "management" becoming a dirty word to many, an important gain for the doctors as they continue to defend the sanctity of their professional autonomy against the encroachments of the administrators. The system for delivering health care in the NHS therefore continues to be desperately short of the incentives needed to maximise efficiency in the use of its most valuable resource — the skills of its doctors and nurses.

One area where the Conservative Government after 1979 joined battle with the established forces within the NHS — and where it must continue to battle — is in the arrangements for the provision of cleaning, catering and laundry services for hospitals. These ancillary services were traditionally provided "in-house" by direct employees of the health service. We took the view, however, that they were likely to be provided more economically and probably to a higher standard by private contractors. We saw a useful parallel in our moves against the wasteful Direct Labour Organisations of local authorities.

There is much evidence that the quality of the ancillary services in the NHS hospitals had been declining for years although, inevitably, it is largely anecdotal. Many people with long experience in the service have told me how they have endured falling standards over the years — dirty wards, badly washed laundry and poor food — as the discipline and commitment of the workers has declined and trade union militancy has increased. It would be possible to dismiss such views as the usual nostalgia for a past which never existed but a number of scandals which did emerge into public view suggest strongly that in all too many cases they were likely to be correct. The most outrageous case which came to light was that of the Stanley Royd Hospital in Wakefield. 29 people were killed by food poisoning and the subsequent inquiry revealed an alarming history of slackness by the catering staff and the failure of management to exert control.

Despite this record, even in this area the NHS has proved extraordinarily resistant to change — an experience which has further discouraged politicians from attempting the very much more fundamental reforms that are needed. In the first round of battle the proposal to privatise the ancillary services, following the precedent of the direct labour organisations of the local authorities, was watered down to the concept of "competitive tendering", so that the existing in-house employees could compete on equal terms with private contractors.

The proposition seems entirely reasonable; the difficulty was in establishing anything like equal terms. The great majority of health authorities were extremely reluctant to upset the *status quo* and were opposed to the introduction of outside contractors. General managers were, with every justification, apprehensive about the difficulties they would encounter in any change-over and the trade unions and other spokesmen of the in-house workers did everything they could to feed these apprehensions. Faced with the resistance of both managers and workers, reinforced in many cases by their own convictions that privatisation would be wrong, many (perhaps most) health authority members were ready to ensure that the in-house bids were given favourable treatment once the process of competitive tendering was forced upon them. It is also fair to record that the process had a very salutary psychological effect on the in-house workers, for example in their work practices and pay bargaining.

However, many devices were used to frighten off potential bidders for the contracts from the private sector or, if they failed, to ensure that the in-house bid appeared to be the most acceptable (if not necessarily the lowest — for example in the way that in-house redundancy payments would be calculated). And among the small minority of cases where contracts have actually been awarded to outside contractors, their performance has been subjected to the most intense and often hostile scrutiny and their shortcomings, real or imagined, loudly publicised. So much ingenuity was displayed that it is worthy of a separate study of its own but it will suffice here to say that the exercise in seeking to introduce competition into the provision of ancillary services has provided a classic demonstration of the deeply unsatisfactory nature of the NHS structure. It was instructive for me, as the Minister responsible, to learn the extent to which I had to resort to cajolery to implement the policy. When the duly elected government, bearing full financial and political responsibility for the NHS, sought to introduce a change which it believed, with much justification, would release more public money for the treatment of patients it was faced with a long and determined rearguard action by the service which made Sir John Moore's retreat to Corunna look like instant surrender.

The net result of the competitive tendering initiative has been similar to other attempts to introduce reforms into the NHS — significant political damage and relatively little to show for it. After some four years of effort about 80% of services had been put out to tender and only one in six had been awarded the private sector. It was claimed that the process had created savings of just under £100 million, but my own experience of the failure of health authorities to ensure that in-house tenderers perform to the standards promised in their contract bids leads me to believe that in practice even this disappointing total will not be realised.

A similar fate met the Conservative Government's effort to dispose of land and property owned by the NHS but which was surplus to its real needs. An official study suggested that this could realise funds of at least £170 million and possibly "as much as £750 million if full advantage were taken of the development potential of certain properties", together with various other substantial savings.[1] However, the harsh reality (or should it be unreality?) of British health politics quickly intervened to dampen such optimism. An effective campaign was mounted alleging that the Government intended to "throw the nurses on to the streets" and the Secretary of State, Norman Fowler, retreated in considerable disorder so that the expectations of savings have been massively scaled down.

We also strongly urged health authorities to look for opportunities to develop their own sources of income, for example by providing additional services for hospital patients and their visitors. A number of managers responded very positively to this challenge and many innovations have been introduced, such as hiring out unwanted sites for retail shops or leasing space in waiting areas for advertising videos. Inevitably, of course, there have been objections to the introduction of commerce into the temples of the NHS and the Addenbrooke Hospital at Cambridge, for example, was obliged to abandon a scheme to provide photographs of newly-born babies and their parents. There have been many complaints that hospitals should concentrate exclusively on treating their patients rather than generating additional income — and, in any case, such schemes could only provide an extremely small addition to hospital finances. After the intensification of the NHS crisis in November 1987, these "income generation" initiatives were given another boost by Health Ministers, who hoped that they would achieve savings of some £20 million in the year.

The "cost improvements" to be achieved by better management and the savings produced by competitive tendering and the sale of NHS real estate were all sensible initiatives. However, even on the most optimistic estimate they could never generate more than about £200 million a year at best, a figure which, welcome though it is, has to be set against NHS spending of over £20,000 million and against the political bloodletting involved. It comes nowhere near to solving the resource pressures on health spending.

Despite these experiences, the power of the NHS myth continues to be so potent that governments will continue to search for salvation *within* Aneurin Bevan's framework and a number of ideas, most of them not new, are in the air.

One old favourite is the idea of "hotel charges" for stays in hospitals, considered and rejected in the past by such disparate Ministers as Richard Crossman and Keith Joseph — and in December, 1987 by Margaret Thatcher. For many years we have had the anomaly that the elderly lose part of their state retirement pension after they have been in hospital for six weeks but the rest of us are asked to pay nothing for our keep however long we are in hospital. The resistance of the service to the imposition of a charging system has always been based on the assertion that its cost of administration could not be justified by the money raised at a level of charges which would be regarded as tolerable. This somewhat circular argument has been strengthened as modern techniques and methods have led in recent years to a steady reduction in the average length of stay in hospital.

As the professionals within the service have, in recent years, moved a little nearer to understanding that the solution to the problems of the NHS can no longer be found in using the political advantages given to them by the system to squeeze ever more money out of the Treasury, they have been forced to turn their minds to the challenge of using more effectively the resources that are available. To make any headway in this direction the NHS will need to embrace a concept which, as we have seen, was ignored by its founders and which it resisted for decades — that treatments could, and certainly should, be costed before any sensible judgements can be made about the allocation of necessarily limited resources.

With excruciating slowness against experienced and determined opposition, some progress in this area is now being made. The Korner Committee reported in 1983 on the need for the NHS to introduce modern cost information systems and the essence of their proposals are now being implemented. The resistance of the medical profession to the idea of "clinical budgetting" is at last showing some signs of weakening, although many battles have yet to be fought. The massive differences in the productivity of individual hospital consultants suggest strongly that this is an area where extremely expensive and scarce resources could be much better used.

There is a growing interest in the scope for developing an "internal market" within the confines of the NHS structure, which has always been so ruinously deficient of incentives to efficiency. An early advocate in this field was the American academic, Alain C. Enthoven, whose 1985 essay *Reflections on the Management of the National Health Service* attracted considerable attention from specialists. Enthoven was at pains to make clear, however, that his paper was based "on the assumption that proposals for radical change in the NHS, such as conversion to an insurance scheme, are wholly unrealistic. I do not sense any real demand for such a change.'[2] After more years of bitter experience, however, that assumption is much less valid than it was and the objective of this book is to make the idea of change in the NHS become more realistic.

The essence of the proposals to introduce an internal market into the NHS is that there should be a major reform of the arrangements for cross-charging between health authorities so that each authority should be able to buy services directly, either from other authorities or from the private sector. Every District Health Authority would receive a *per capita* revenue and capital allowance for each resident, based on the existing RAWP formula (i.e. related to historic spending and future needs).

Any device which would improve the use of NHS resources and

would be likely to reduce hospital waiting lists deserves very careful and favourable consideration. Inevitably, however, there are serious snags. The present right of GP's to refer their patients to a consultant of their choice would be restricted. Disparities in patient care between Districts would be inescapable and Ministers would be embroiled in the ensuing controversies but with little or no power to intervene actively. There would be a non-stop battle with the Government on the size of the *per capita* allowance to be paid to particular districts. Most fundamental of all, it would do nothing to increase the total of resources committed to health care in Britain.

There are two other areas of research in the field of health economics which deserve to be considered, both for their own sake as a means of educating NHS professionals to a more effective use of resources and for the contribution they might make to the evolution of an internal market in health services.

The University of York and the North Western Regional Health Authority have in recent years been working on the concept of Quality Adjusted Life-Years or QALY's. The object is to combine the measurement of QALY's with the available data on treatment cost to provide a new and more valuable criterion to be used in the allocation of health resources.

It is an arcane area of study and there are many problems to be overcome. For example, the main trailblazer of this effort, Professor Alan Maynard, has pointed to one expert who argues that 10% of health care actually harms patients' health and therefore reduces QALY's while another 10% has a neutral effect. He also emphasises the very poor levels of evaluation of health care therapies in current use, with little comparison of alternative methods of treatment or of no treatment at all. Nevertheless, despite these difficulties and the fact that an element of subjective judgement is probably inescapable, this work is surely of great potential value and has already produced some interesting results. For example, using this method of evaluation Maynard shows that one QALY from a hip replacement costs less than one twentieth of a QALY from a renal dialysis, whilst another study from the

University of York shows that a kidney transplant is, in these terms, likely to be nearly ten times more cost-effective than an increasingly popular treatment known as CAPD — Continuous Ambulatory Peritoneal Dialysis ("portable" dialysis). Even if these procedures become accepted, of course, there will remain the terrible problem of making decisions on "cost-effectiveness" related to human lives. Essentially, this is something that doctors have always done. Maynard and his supporters maintain that their techniques will enable doctors to reach their decisions on the basis of more complete and reliable criteria. It is a matter of judgement and priorities which fundamentally, in one form or another, no health system can avoid; the NHS has merely succeeded, at least for a time, in giving the illusion of being able to do so.

Another system designed to control health costs which is now under close scrutiny in a number of countries is the concept of "diagnosis-related groups" (DRG's) which was embodied in legislation passed by the United States Congress in 1983. This is a mechanism for identifying particular medical problems and establishing a scale of payment for their treatment. The Americans have produced a list of 470 DRG's and the French Government is looking hard at the idea. The Belgians adopted a similar system some years ago but ran into trouble with their medical profession over the level of fees to be paid, leading to a national doctors' strike. Problems have also developed in the United States with hospitals and doctors seeking to cheat in claiming DRG payments — maintaining, for example, that they have treated two conditions rather than just one.

These are all ways of trying to make the money made available for the NHS go round further and faster. As such they would all deserve to be encouraged were it not for two facts of crucial and over-riding importance: firstly, none of them will lead to any significant increase in the *total* of resources available and that is essential; secondly, they will be seized upon as potential lifebelts by governments and others who do not wish or are too scared to face up to the realities of forty years of the National Health Service; they will become pretexts for further prevarication.

This chapter has discussed possible ways of making the NHS straitjacket a little more comfortable. Politicians still desperately hoping to avoid facing up to reality see yet one more possibility. They believe we might be able to slip painlessly out of the straitjacket altogether as a steadily rising percentage of the population signs up for private medical insurance.

I believe there is no such possibility, even if the government sought to hasten the process by income tax concessions.

It is true that for a few years after the Conservative victory in 1979 there was a substantial rise in private spending on health. Even so, it still represents only about 6% of what is spent on the NHS, the increase having stablised in the mid-1980's. About 10% of the population are now covered by private insurance arrangements for *hospital* treatment and, as the economy grows, it seems reasonable to expect a modest rise in that figure. However, unless the trends change dramatically, it will be very many years before it reaches anywhere near 25% — the sort of level at which those who cling to the hope that this phenomenon offers the escape route believe significant and relatively painless reforms in the NHS could be achieved.

Experience shows that increases in private health spending do not seem to act as a brake on the growing pressures on the NHS and that demand for it has actually been greater in those parts of the country where *per capita* spending on the NHS is higher. If suspicions grew that the government was relying on the expansion of private health insurance to resolve the dilemma of NHS funding there would certainly be a long and very bitter political battle. The "two-tier" and the "North-South" banners would be unfurled with a vengeance.

We cannot, for much longer, survive within the straitjacket. Nor can we slip out of it painlessly, as we shall be forced to conclude when we take amore comprehensive look at the possible options in a subsequent chapter. There is no easy answer available: that is the lesson of the last forty years.

7

How Much Does the
Health Service "Need"?

There is one issue on which there is almost total unanimity in Britain: the great majority believe that we ought to be spending more on health care. Even the "driest" of us in the Conservative Party, who have insisted for years that our economy can only be restored to vitality when the burden of state spending is reduced to something nearer that borne by other Western countries — and can now point to Britain's recent experience to support our case — have accepted this. Hence in every Budget speech and Autumn Statement made by whichever Chancellor of the Exchequer and in every Whitehall battle on public expenditure, exceptional priority is always given to health spending. As the economy has grown in recent years, the resources devoted to the NHS have grown more rapidly.

Yet, as concern about the service has grown at the same time as spending has increased dramatically in real terms, a school of thought (in some cases that may be a charitable term) has developed which maintains that all would be well if only, perhaps buttressed by a few organisational changes, the Government found a little more money for health. "We're nearly there, just another £200 million or so", says the General Secretary of the Royal College of Nursing — who presumably must realise he is talking of an increase of something like one per cent in a budget which grew by over 30% in eight years (as the chorus of despair swelled).

This is a classic British paradox, with some of those who were loudest in their complaints about the "underfunding" of the NHS now saying they do not want as much money as is spent in many European countries. The explanation is to be found largely in their determination to maintain — or fear of trying to change — the *status quo* and their dawning realisation that European levels of spending would inevitably involve changes they do not even wish to contemplate.

Some of the protagonists of this school point to the inefficiences remaining in the NHS, in particular the dearth of costing and incentive mechanisms in the use of clinical and medical resources. They also maintain that complaints about a shortage of nurses in Britain are unjustified, quoting the fact that "there are 85 nurses for 100,000 Britons compared with 50 in America, 45 in France and 35 in West Germany." (*The Economist* 12th December, 1987).

Both points are valid and certainly, as I stress elsewhere in this book, we need to eliminate those inefficiences which forty years of attempted reform of the NHS have failed to remove. On balance, however, we have created a health service which has low overheads by international standards (see Chapter Six, pages 86-87) and it is quite unrealistic to believe that with just a little more money and a little more "efficiency" difficult decisions can be avoided.

What these minimalist reformers and those who, incredibly, still cling to the hope that the National Health crisis will somehow go away of its own accord do not seem prepared to recognise is the power of some of the other pressures building up *within* the service. There are time bombs which will soon explode unless they are defused by radical action. These are the pressures caused by the low pay which has been a feature of most parts of the National Health Service since it started (with some significant exceptions, notably many London hospital consultants). Whether or not there is a return to the industrial militancy which was such an ugly feature of the NHS in the '70's and played a major part in the defeat of the Labour Government in May 1979, poor pay scales are already causing serious staffing problems in many areas and these problems are bound to get worse. For example, in many parts of the country it is becoming increasingly difficult for the NHS to compete with the private sector and recruit and retain the secretaries, especially those with medical experience, who are vital to the efficient operation of hospitals.

The growing shortage of nurses is a much more politically lethal time bomb, for the reasons we have already discussed. Although the substantial pay increases and the reductions in working hours introduced by the Conservative Government after 1979 resulted in the recruitment of over 60,000 more nurses, shortages are acute and growing. It is becoming particularly difficult to recruit nurses to work in the intensive care units of some of the leading hospitals in London and some of the other major cities — where such problems can be guaranteed to attract the maximum public attention and therefore cause the greatest political embarrassment.

Some estimates show that if we are to restore the establishment of nurses to levels which would be considered adequate by traditional NHS standards we shall need 50% of all girls *leaving school with at least five good GCSE's to become nurses* — a very unlikely prospect. Campaigning by the Royal College of Nursing for further improvements in the training, status and working conditions of nurses — as, for example, in their Project 2000 — will exacerbate still further this highly explosive situation.

Other expensive trouble has also been stored up in recent years as hospitals have cut back on their maintenance budgets in order to meet staff costs which have been rising faster than the increases in funding they have received. Whilst guilty of some hyperbole, Dr Tony Smith, Deputy Editor of the *British Medical Journal*, was not far wrong when he complained, in the issue of 2nd January 1988, that "virtually every hospital is dirty and many are filthy; many are unpainted, unrepaired and unmaintained."

Dr Smith warned that the NHS was moving towards "terminal decline" and pointed to the glaring disparities in health spending between Britain and other European countries. Citing figures expressed in US dollars per head, he put UK expenditure at 493, the Netherlands 828, France 853, Germany 1,000 and Switzerland 1,111. Dr Smith, who does not appear to belong to the minimalist school to which I referred earlier, did not go on to point out that all the other countries he listed funded their health spending through a variety of insurance arrangements rather than a government-financed scheme on the British model.

There is a mass of evidence which demonstrates how the NHS has, for decades, failed to meet the demand — and the reasonable "needs" — of the British people. The most glaring and quantifiable indicator is, of course, the scandal of the huge waiting lists for hospital treatment. This is a phenomenon virtually unknown in other advanced countries but we have become accustomed to a national queue of between half and three quarters of a million people waiting to get into our hospitals and for many of us to suffer years of unnecessary pain before being treated.

Of all the democratic nations, surely only the British would have tolerated such a situation for so long? It is the ultimate demonstration of the power of the NHS myth which we have allowed to be exercised over us.

The number of doctors and hospital beds is another, easily quantifiable, means of international comparison of the levels of health services provision and here, again, Britain scores badly. I take below the countries listed by Dr Smith as spending (from all sources) more than we do on health:

	U.K.	Nether-lands	France	Ger-many	Switzer-land
Doctors (per 10,000)	16	19	17	23	25
Hospital beds (do.)	87	122	111	114	127

(Source: *Universities Work for Health*[1])

Academic studies over many years have shown how the NHS has failed to deliver to the British people the standards of medical care enjoyed by other advanced countries with different health systems. These facts are well known to NHS insiders but not to the great majority who have continued to cling to their faith in Bevan's creation of 1948.

For example, the *Health: The Politician's Dilemma*, published by the Office of Health Economics, shows a table for the acceptance rates for end-stage renal failure in nine European countries in 1984. Top of the list was Belgium, with 67.8 per million, and Britain was bottom, with 35.9. Even Spain did better, with 54.3.[2]

In an essay in *Health Care UK 1984*, Robert Maxwell reported that "people are going without treatment, whereas they would receive it in much of Europe or North America. In examples such as megavolt radiation therapy, treatment for end-stage renal failure, scanning and coronary by-pass surgery, the UK is consistently at the low end of the scale of provision (see *Advanced and Expensive Medical Technology*, EEC, 1982).[3]

In *The Painful Prescription: Rationing Hospital Care*, Henry Aaron and William Schwartz pointed to many deficiencies in the NHS. "Only one-tenth to one-fifth the number of intensive care beds available per capita as in the United States" ... "the British have the capacity to perform only a fifth as many (CT) scans per capita as do Americans" ... "a technology now recognised as a powerful, indeed revolutionary, diagnostic tool in many clinical situations". Whilst recognising that the American rate of coronary artery surgery might be too high, they suggested that the fact that in Britain we achieved only 10% of the American level "calls out for an explanation". They noted that "if Britain dialyzed at the same rate as the United States, it would have to increase its total health expenditures by over 1 percent".[4]

A study which brought home to a much wider British public the differences in the levels of provision in other countries appeared in the *Sunday Times* on 6th December 1987. This report compared the experiences of two middle-aged men who had recently suffered heart attacks. The Briton was treated at the Bristol Royal Infirmary and the German at the Robert Bosch Hospital in Stuttgart. The reporter had chosen these two hospitals because they were of similar size and both had cardiac surgery units.

This illuminating and powerful article should have convinced any reader that the fact the Germans spend over twice as much on health *does* provide them with significantly better services. The difference cannot merely be explained away by the extravagance of the German system or the higher salaries of German doctors and other health workers.

The reporters were immediately struck by the waiting list phenomenon. "At Bristol, 2,431 people were waiting for treatment, many for surgery such as hip replacements, some for major heart operations or pace-makers. There are 205 people waiting for cardiac surgery — 26 for more than a year. At Robert Bosch, however, as at other West German hospitals, waiting lists are virtually unheard of."

Bristol was said to be in the grip of a cash crisis, with two wards and an operating theatre temporarily closed, cardiologists told to fit only 90 pacemakers before April 1988 rather than the 130 they wanted to do and patients sent home as soon as possible so that their beds could be stripped and reoccupied within an hour. Whilst "at the privately-owned, non-profit making Bosch Hospital, such financial problems are, so far, unthinkable."

Both operations were successful but the Englishman had been waiting for his for 15 months after his heart attack and was sent home after a week. The German was held in hospital to recuperate for three weeks and was then sent for six weeks of convalescence at a health spa on the shores of a Bavarian lake.

It is true that the article, rightly, indicates that German health spending is also under pressure but the overwhelming impression is of a level of care far beyond British standards. And the same situation applies in other European countries. We must now try to put a figure on what we probably need to spend to bring our service up to somewhere near the same level.

To find an answer to that conundrum we need to have recourse to the international statistics which are available although in using them *it is crucial to understand the great difficulty of obtaining data which are circulated on exactly the same basis in each country.*

The absolutist defenders of Bevan's creation regularly point out the now massive gap between the level of health spending in Britain and most other Western countries but the fact they resolutely ignore is that it began to develop only after the NHS was launched. In 1950 we spent 3.9% of our GNP on health compared with, for example, 3.4% in both France and Sweden (recognising the caveat entered above about the use of such statistics). Even in Canada and the United States spending was only at 4.0% and 4.5% respectively. Since then, of course, the position has been transformed. As most Western countries achieved faster rates of growth than Britain, at least until the last few years, the *proportion* of their increasing wealth devoted to health care also rose.

By 1985 — on the basis of the latest statistics available — among the industrialised nations only Italy and Ireland spent less on health, in *per capita* terms, than we did. By then health spending in France had risen to 8.6% of GNP and in Sweden to 8.8%. Germany was spending 9.2% and the United States 10.5%. In Britain we spent only 5.9%.

It is clear that as countries become more prosperous, they tend to devote an increasing proportion of their wealth to health spending. But the explanation of this gap which has appeared between Britain and other industrialised nations must be attributed, in large measure, to the differences in our health systems. The NHS is a closed system; the insurance-based schemes chosen by other countries are much better able to facilitate and encourage private spending on health care which supplements what it is possible to provide with state funding.

Some defenders of the NHS suggest that much of the difference in health spending can be accounted for by the higher cost of living and wages which obtain in other countries. The statistician's way round this problem is to make comparisons on the basis of "purchasing power parities". The table opposite uses this method and shows how substantial is the real gap between Britain and other countries and how it widened between 1970 and 1984.

A recent IMF study has confirmed that differences in health spending cannot — at least to any significant extent — be accounted for by differences in general wage levels. In fact, hourly earnings in Britain are higher (11.00 Swiss Francs) than in France (8.55) or Sweden (9.81). Earnings in Germany are 12.09 SF.[5]

The latest available figures show that in 1984 a selection of fifteen OECD countries, including Britain, Ireland and Italy, spent an

Per Capita Health Spending (US$ at GDP PPP's, current prices)

	1970	1984
United Kingdom	161	658
France	223	1,145
Germany	220	1,079
Netherlands	232	1,011
Sweden	359	1,445
United States	366	1,637

(Source: OECD 1987, table 20)

average of 9.2% of their GNP on their health services. We spent 5.9%[6]. It is therefore entirely reasonable to conclude that, if we are to produce standards of care which approach those of comparable countries, we also need to spend about 9% of our GDP.

In other words, we should be looking for a system which would generate an increase in health spending in this country of some 50%. In terms of the 1987-88 NHS budget this implies additional spending of over *£10 billion.*

On the basis of per capita spending this would still leave us significantly behind other European countries. Using the figures quoted by Dr Smith in the British Medical Journal (page 98 of this Chapter) it would imply an increase in British spending from US$493 to $739, which would still be well short of the Netherlands (828), France (853), Germany (1,000) or Switzerland (1,111). In the light of the evidence I have cited above on differences in health care standards, efficiency, cost of living and incomes, an increase of this magnitude in health spending in Britain could not be represented as unreasonable.

The problem is that no Chancellor of the Exchequer of any political persuasion would be able — nor should be willing — to contemplate increasing his spending on health to anywhere near that level, which would be far above that of any other Western government. It would either involve massive and unacceptable raids on other spending programmes — the only areas which could produce those sort of savings are social security, education or defence — or an increase in total government expenditure which would have malign and far-reaching consequences for the whole economy.

To find this sum for the NHS would, if the savings were found in one Department, mean slashing education or defence spending by more than half, with predictable political and international consequences. In practice, in the very unlikely event that any government would be mad enough to embark on such a course, an attempt would be made to spread the misery of spending cuts over many Departments — with a resultant amplification of the political mayhem that would follow.

The effect of accommodating this rise in the NHS budget by simply adding it to the total of government spending would be even more disastrous. On the basis of the 1987/88 figures, this would represent an increase in public expenditure of 6.5% and the reversal of the policy which has been the foundation of our economic success in recent years — that whilst government spending is allowed to rise in real terms it should fall as a proportion of national income, at least until it approaches levels regarded as normal in other developed economies. Such an increase in public spending, taking it back to some 44% of GDP, would, rightly, be interpreted as signalling a return to the fiscal irresponsibility of Labour's worst years, with all the inescapable consequences of loss of international confidence, depreciation of sterling, inflation, high interest rates and a precipitate return to the spiral of economic decline from which we have so recently escaped. Very soon we should be back to cuts in the health service even more severe than Mr Dennis Healey was obliged to impose when he was bailed out by the International Monetary Fund in 1976. A very vicious circle indeed.

Leaving aside, for the purposes of discussion, the economic impact of bringing *government* spending on health up to the level of 9% of GNP — a luxury which, in real life, we should not be permitted — there would be other negative aspects of such a policy.

It would do nothing at all to remove the provision of health care from its position at the hottest part of the political cauldron, a situation which has hamstrung the development of modern services in this country. Indeed, things would get worse. The allocation 9% of our GNP on health, however well administered, would certainly not relieve all pressures for still more spending, as the experience of other countries demonstrates. Having scored such a major advance, the appetite of the NHS professionals and their confidence in the political power at their command would grow and so their demands on the Exchequer would not abate. Their clamour would still be heard above the outraged squeals of the other spending Departments and their defenders.

The increase in spending would do nothing to improve the fundamental structural weaknesses of the NHS which we looked at in Chapter Five. We should still have the fuzzy relationships and built-in conflicts between Health Ministers and the NHS and its Regions, and between health authority chairmen, members, managers and professionals which exists at present and which forty years of efforts, including the proposals of Sir Roy Griffiths, have failed to resolve.

And, above all, we should still be inflicted with the pressures generated by a service which aims to be "free at the point of treatment", pressures suffered by the health services of no other industrialised country.

I hope and believe that however strong may be our lingering *emotional* attachment to the NHS, the logic of the foregoing has brought us to the following set of conclusions:

* the particular package of arrangements for providing a comprehensive system of health care which, after a generation of national debate, was finally chosen by Aneurin Bevan, no longer meets modern needs. Indeed, it was inherently flawed from the beginning, even though it has many achievements to its credit, particularly as an *emergency* service, and has generated a remarkable degree of dedication from many of those who work in it and loyalty from the general public.

* whilst it has devoured an ever-larger proportion of public expenditure and national wealth, the NHS has proved increasingly unable to cope with the rising pressures generated by an

ageing population, advancing technology and higher expectations of the consumer. We are falling ever further behind the levels of health care now regarded as normal by other industrialised countries. The solutions already tried or under consideration — better management, cost improvements, competitive tendering, sale of real estate, income generation, internal markets and the rest — offer no prospect of providing the level of additional funding that is "needed".

* The most useful guide to the level of health spending we "ought" to have in this country is probably provided by the experience of other Western countries, who tend to spend around 9% of their GNP's (which in many cases are higher than ours in *per capita* terms) — but much less of it is *government* spending. To match this would require a 50% increase in the NHS budget under the existing system — a rise which no British government would contemplate as it would have disastrous consequences for the rest of the public sector and for the economy as a whole.

* We therefore need to develop a system which would generate substantial new funding for our health services — and preferably one which would eliminate or at least significantly reduce the other weaknesses of the NHS that we have identified.

The principal objective of this book is to get the country to accept these conclusions and to take forward a national debate on what now needs to be done. It must be a much more open, less emotional and better informed debate than we have had for the last forty years between the NHS insiders and the politicians. With very few exceptions, the insiders have been content to work within the existing system, regarding it as a mechanism to extract even larger amounts from the public purse, whilst often defending their own particular corners against attempts to achieve a more sensible use of resources. The politicians have played the same game when out of office and when in office have tried by every hook and crook to make the funding they have squeezed out of the Treasury go even further.

The time for this fudging and first aid is now over. The NHS Emperor has no clothes, or at least not enough of them to be respectable, and, as a nation, we should now be realistic and honest enough to recognise the fact.

Of course, the going will be difficult. The wiseacres in every political party will persist in trying to steer well clear of it. Even Margaret Thatcher, cautious underneath her remarkable achievements, until recently regarded the mere contemplation of significant NHS reform as a bridge too far.

Yet it must now happen, if only because it is being forced upon us by the economic and political realities afflicting the service. And as it does, I believe the difficulties will turn out to be much less formidable than they now appear to a nation which has been brainwashed for forty years by professionals with vested interests, superficial leader writers and mesmerized politicians.

Britain is now a very different country from the one which accepted Bevan's recipe in 1946. We have more confidence in ourselves and we have more experience. We have seen that socialism, collectivism and neo-Keynesianism do not work. All the other fashions of the immediate post-war period have been rejected and reversed — nationalisation, public sector housing, politicised trade unions, municipal socialism and the rest. The NHS, which took health care further down the socialist path in Britain than in any other Western country, is the only survivor of that period of political engineering and there is now massive evidence that the time has come when it, too, must be re-appraised.

We are now a society in which the great majority live in their own homes or aspire to do so. There are now nearly as many share-owners as there are members of trade unions. Even the leader of the Labour Party appears now to accept that he cannot say to a docker earning £400 per week, living in his own house with a new car, a video recorder and a time-share holiday home in Spain, that "socialism will rescue you from all this". With this growing affluence has come a rise in the demand for better standards of health care, as has happened in other industrialised countries. We must now find a way to harness that affluence and the rising demand to provide more resources for our health service.

Ironically enough, this search may well not involve turning away entirely from our national experience but rather to going back to ideas that were current *before* Aneurin Bevan pushed his own scheme through the Labour Cabinet in 1946 against the opposition of powerful colleagues such as Herbert Morrison and against the policy which had been approved by the most recent Labour Party Congress.

It may also involve benefiting from the experience of other countries in their efforts to improve the quality of health care — and this is something we shall look at in the next chapter.

But the most important thing of all is that we should now embark on a careful and undogmatic consideration of how we may best provide the improved medical services we shall clearly expect in the years ahead, disregarding the shrill chorus of indignation that the threat of new thinking is bound to unleash.

8
What Can We Learn from Others?

In looking for ways out of our problems, it will clearly make sense to examine the experience of other countries in providing systems of health care. Yet this is an area which has received very little attention in Britain — except from a few specialists in the field, often with their own axes to grind. This insular attitude is yet another manifestation of the power of the NHS myth; clinging ever more desperately to our "envy of the world" illusion, we have not wanted to learn what other countries have been doing lest we might discover they have found better answers than ours.

The sole exception to this general lack of interest in overseas experience has been a readiness of public opinion in this country, duly catered for by the media, to focus on horror stories about health care in the United States. We are happy to read stories from America of the poor being denied medical treatment, of the middle-class being bankrupted by hospital bills and of rapacious doctors piling up their millions. In part they serve to feed the anti-Americanism which is one of the unattractive features of contemporary attitudes in Britain. Their more important function, however, is to provide solace when we contemplate our long hospital waiting lists or any of the other signs of the strains afflicting the NHS.

In fact, this is a misleading and increasingly out-dated representation of the American health scene.

An adequate review of the health care arrangements of the rest of the advanced world would require at least one book and probably several. This chapter must therefore be very selective. It is, nevertheless, possible to point to some general conclusions and observations which are relevant to our theme and our search for better answers to our problems.

The fundamental problems are, of course, the same in every country which enjoys a relatively high standard of living and a democratic system — and, hence, where the voice of the consumer is powerful. They all suffer the same trio of pressures we have become familiar with in Britain: the effects of ageing populations, advancing and more costly medical techniques and rising aspirations to good health. It is not surprising, therefore, that there is concern in virtually every industrialised country about how to contain the relentless increase in the cost of health care and to meet public expectations of high-grade medical cover. As a result, in recent years there has been a good deal of new thinking and experimentation about how to organise and fund health services, providing us with food for both thought and action.

Indeed, it is striking (and depressing) to note how much more — and more significant — new thinking and experimentation there has been overseas than in Britain. It is true that we have had forty years of commissions, reviews and studies of the problems of our health services, as noted in Chapters Four and Five, but they have produced no changes of any substance and our difficulties have deepened remorselessly into the crisis that now confronts us. Our failure to make, or even contemplate, major changes has not been because the NHS does not need them but much more because of the inhibiting effect of the NHS myth. We now have much to learn from the experience of others in the delivery of better quality health care and in the control of costs.

As we have already noted, in the past two decades many countries have outpaced us in their health spending. Even allowing for the fact that NHS administration costs are significantly below those in other advanced countries and that it provides the United Kingdom with an excellent *emergency* service, their citizens enjoy substantially better medical cover than the British. Many indicators could be quoted to justify this assertion and I have already cited a number of them in the previous chapter.

These countries can also boast other advantages. Firstly, those working within the health services tend to be better paid than their counterparts in Britain (where relatively low pay is an important factor in our control of administrative costs). Secondly, they are much more advanced in the introduction into their services of incentives for the efficient use of medical resources. Finally, all of them have evolved systems which have lifted the issue of health care further away from the centre of the political battlefield than is the case in this country.

With the exception of New Zealand, which has already embarked on a major re-think, no advanced country has adopted a health system which replicates the socialistic formula of the National Health Service, being almost totally funded and controlled by central Government. Instead, most have developed systems which are based on concepts carefully examined and, in some areas, put into practice by British governments between 1911 and 1946 but which were then rejected by Bevan in favour of the structure which in essence we still have today, despite forty years of attempts at reform. As we have seen in Chapter Two, the debate during those years was whether a comprehensive health service could best be provided through an insurance-based system or one organised, and probably funded, on a regional or local level. In 1946 it would have been possible to expand the National Health Insurance scheme instituted by Lloyd George in 1911, and which by then covered some 24 million people, to encompass the whole of the population. As experience in other countries has demonstrated, this would have been a much more flexible arrangement than Bevan's solution and would have created the possibility of grafting on to it individual contributions. The regional solution, favoured by many in the Labour Party in 1946 and later, always foundered on the difficulty of establishing local sources of finance.

Most of the other countries have tended to develop either insurance-based or regionally-funded health systems or a mixture of the two. Very few of them have adopted the cardinal principle of the NHS, that treatment should be free for everyone at the point of delivery. Whilst special provisions are made for the poor, the elderly or the chronic sick, the great majority of countries regard it as right and sensible for the individual (or his insurer) to make some contribution.

And having avoided the collectivist path followed by Britain, other industrialised countries have not needed to create the unwieldy and unworkable administrative structure through which British governments have tried to control the NHS and which, as we saw in Chapter Five, has proved so resistant to reform.

None of this is to say that these other countries have no problems in the health field: but their problems *are* less daunting than ours and they are more likely to achieve better (though not Utopian) solutions because of the inherent flexibility of their systems. Let us now look at some of their characteristics.

The American Experience

I have already mentioned the consolation the British tend to find in their bleak image of the American medical system. It is generally regarded as the health service furthest from the NHS on the political spectrum, having the least degree of government intervention while we have the greatest.

In fact public funding plays a larger role in meeting health care costs in the United States than is generally appreciated in this country; when federal, state and local spending are included they accounted for 41% of the total in 1985. Most of this expenditure is taken up by the Medicare and Medicaid programmes, which were introduced in 1965 and produced a sharp increase in the proportion of national resources spent on health. Medicare provides services for those over 65, who numbered nearly 16 million, or about 7% of the total population, at the end of 1983. Three out of five of this group held private health insurance to supplement the benefits available through Medicare. Medicaid is a combined federal-state programme for the poor or near-poor. About 10% of Americans have no health insurance. Some of these are self-employed individuals who choose not to buy it but the great majority are unemployed or in low-wage jobs working for employers who do not pay for medical cover.

Of the remainder, about 80% of Americans are covered by one or more forms of private health plan — leaving 10% or so who work in the public sector — and the majority of them are entitled to benefits of $250,000 or more. The cover is provided by the Blue Cross or Blue Shield plans, commercial insurance companies or by independent plans.

The horror stories about American medicine which we enjoy so much are often exaggerated and out-dated — but there can be no denying that they contain a considerable basis of truth. There are many elements in the American experience which, as we look for ways to improve health care in Britain, provide us with examples to avoid. The plight of the uninsured and the indigent can be very difficult indeed in the USA if they fall sick. Cuts in federal spending on Medicaid have passed a larger share of the burden on to the states and local governments, whose resources have often proved inadequate. In the past, it had been the practice of many community hospitals to provide care for those who could not pay and recover their costs from surcharges on the bills of paying patients and insurers. As increasing pressures have squeezed profit margins all round, this practice has become less common so that the community hospitals — unless life-threatening emergencies are involved — now usually refer poor patients to the overcrowded and underfunded public hospitals run by local governments.

The explosion in American health costs, caused by the considerable degree of freedom to set their prices enjoyed by the providers, the power of the American medical profession and the open-ended subsidies to Medicare and Medicaid, inevitably afflicted the insured majority. One Blue Cross executive told me that in the 1950s a family could buy their most comprehensive contract for some $110 a year. By the early 80s, family cover cost $3,000 a year.

For some two decades American health costs grew at about 12% a year. By 1965 they accounted for 6.2% of the GNP — which included a sharp jump on the introduction of Medicare and Medicaid — but by 1984 this figure had risen to 10.6%, despite the fact that the economy had grown at a formidable rate over the period.

These are some of the negative aspects of the American experience, which blind and unreasoning defenders of the NHS are fond of quoting. Certainly, they should not be ignored but we should also be readier to look at what the Americans have achieved, particularly in recent years. Firstly, there can be little challenge to the primacy of American medicine on the international stage. Whilst individual specialists and units in the United Kingdom, Germany, Japan and other countries may claim to be among the world leaders in their particular field, the all-round excellence of American medicine and research transcends merely the size of the country or its economy. As a consequence, citizens of the United States have, in general, access to better and more effective health care than those of any other country.

The response to the steep rise in American health costs, aggravated recently by a second explosion — this time in court awards in medical damage claims and hence in liability insurance premia — has been the emergence of a range of innovatory schemes and devices. A number of them show signs of being successful and some, at least, could well have lessons for Britain.

In 1983 the United States federal government amended the Social Security Act so that payments under the Medicare programme would no longer be on a fee-for-service basis paid retro-actively but on a fixed price per case based on diagnosis. Rates were established for each of 467 diagnosis-related groups (DRGs). Independent bodies were established to advise both the Administration and Congress on the annual increase in the DRG rates paid to hospitals which would be needed to take account of changes in various medical and economic factors. In subsequent years, however, substantially lower increases were authorised in most instances.

This fixed-price approach is now increasingly adopted in the private sector of American medicine and some states have actually passed legislation requiring all third party payers, including Blue Cross and Blue Shield, to use DRGs. Many believe that it is providing a generally effective means of containing costs and is clearly a technique that ought to be beneficial to the NHS, in which, thanks largely to the resistance of the medical profession, there is a lamentable ignorance of the cost of particular treatments.

As with most improvements, there are some drawbacks about the DRG methodology which need to be considered. There are reports, for example, that some hospitals and doctors have found a way round the cost control by claiming to have carried out two treatments, and therefore two DRG payments, when there was only one. Probably the most serious difficulty with the DRG system is that it could deter the introduction of new technology. For example, suppose scientists developed a new prosthetic device to be used in hip replacement surgery which would be a permanent implant whereas the existing technology needs to be replaced, say, every five years. The new device would be likely to be more costly and the DRG rate would be set on the old method. Although the innovation would be cheaper in the long run and provide the patient with better service, the DRG would point to the use of the old technology. A degree of flexibility and imagination will therefore always be needed.

American insurers have, in addition, been exploring a variety of other ways to contain costs — spurred on by employers, who now pay the greater share of the cost of the health insurance of their employees and often of their dependents as well. The rapid escalation of their health insurance bills has threatened the very survival of some companies.

One line of attack, designed to check unjustified demands for medical and other services from individuals enjoying comprehensive medical cover, has been to withdraw the 100% liability of the insurer. This can result in the insured paying a fixed sum or a fixed percentage (usually 20%) of any medical bill he incurs or meeting medical costs of up to, say, $200 a year, before the insurance cover takes effect. These cost-sharing arrangements are known as co-payments.

Employers and insurers are also developing "managed care" schemes. In essence, these are traditional insurances linked to an arrangement which seeks to ensure that the services provided are only those that do what needs to be done at the least cost consistent with *appropriate* care. There is usually provision for co-payments by the insured. Treatment as a hospital in-patient will only be paid for if approved by the insurer's representative, usually a registered nurse. Length of stay in a hospital is specified according to the diagnosis and any extension must be approved by the insurer.

The most prominent feature of American medicine in recent years has been the growth in Health Maintenance Organisations (HMOs). As recorded by David Green in his stimulating review of the history of American health care entitled *Challenge to the NHS*[1], the first HMO was established in Los Angeles in 1929 but until the 1970s and the pressures generated by rising costs, the movement was stifled by the hostility of the medical profession.

An HMO is a self-contained system for providing and funding health care which assumes primary responsibility for maintaining the health of its members. It seeks to do this by managing the health care needs of each member with special emphasis on health education, the prevention of illness and the promotion of sensible lifestyles. It provides a broad range of services in return for a single fee, usually paid monthly, and encourages doctors to provide patients only with the services and treatments which are truly necessary and appropriate.

There are at least four different types of HMO and new arrangements are regularly being introduced as more experience is gained.

One version is known as the *staff model*. All the personnel employed, including the doctors, are salaried and most can earn performance incentives. They work from modern clinics from which they provide most medical and other minor services, together with health education, pre-natal training and nutritional advice. Only complex cases are referred to outside specialists or institutions. In negotiating contracts with hospitals and other providers, the HMO is usually able to obtain favourable rates.

The staff model HMO has been shown to be particularly effective in controlling unnecessary in-patient treatment in hospital, especially for the elderly. One Blue Cross HMO in Massachusetts has reported that with one group of 3,000 randomly-selected over 65s it was able to reduce the number of days spent in hospital by no less than 55% within a very short period. The federal government was so impressed that it made a grant of $500,000 to enable Blue Cross to expand the programme.

One disadvantage of the staff model HMO for the Americans is that it involves relatively heavy investment at the outset. Each medical centre costs several million dollars from which, at the most, only about 30,000 members of the scheme can be serviced. To obtain the best results, for which the recruitment of high-grade doctors and nurses is essential, experience has shown that the HMO needs a population base of between 300,000 and 400,000 within a 25 mile radius. These criteria would be met in Britain's inner cities where the level and quality of services provided by general practitioners tends to be low and the demand for hospital services particularly high.

Another version of the HMO is the *group model*. Under this arrangement the HMO is the corporate legal entity which contracts with an independent, and usually pre-existing, group of doctors, paying them a fixed fee per HMO member each month. The doctors, some of whom will themselves by specialists, are responsible for all admissions to hospitals, with which special rates are negotiated. Not surprisingly, this type of arrangement has been less successful than the staff model HMO in reducing the admission rates to hospitals. Tensions also develop as schemes become well-established and the doctors' group seeks to operate independently of the HMO — creating an element of competition which should benefit the general public. A variation of the group HMO is the *network model*, under which the HMO contracts with more than one independent group practice.

The version of the HMO which has been growing most rapidly in recent years has been the *independent practice association* (IPA). This is an arrangement whereby the HMO contracts with a list of doctors who are practising independently or in groups. It tends to produce the sort of doctor-patient relationships we are accustomed to (and generally favour) in Britain but, whether the contracts are based on capitation payments or fee-for-service, the HMO will always devise arrangements to provide incentives for the doctors to restrict hospital admissions only to those cases where it is properly justified. Under some IPA schemes, community hospitals and their medical staffs are contracted into the HMO, so that the general practitioner, the hospital and the HMO all share a common interest in delivering adequate medical care in the most economical form.

In 1972 5.3 million Americans were enrolled in 142 HMO schemes. By 1985 those figures had increased to 19 million in 431 schemes, with the rate of growth gathering strong momentum in recent years. There is a considerable diversity in their methods and their effectiveness and, certainly, they have their critics, especially among the medical profession where there is resentment at the success of HMOs in bringing costs under better control. These doctors complain that the HMO approach creates incentives to *under*-provide medical services but a number of studies, which all show that the HMOs contain costs significantly better than fee-for-service arrangements, provide no evidence to support this charge. For example Harold Luft,[2] whose approach to the subject seems to have been balanced and objective, concluded: "But one who expected HMOs to skimp on quality in order to cut costs would find little evidence to support that contention." The fact is that it is in the interests of the HMO to avoid a situation in which the subscriber will need expensive and extensive treatment and hospitalisation. There is therefore an incentive to provide preventive health care, tests and investigations when necessary and good quality primary care. Above all, the principal protection of the individual is that if he is not satisfied with the service he is being given, he is able to take his custom elsewhere. The general lesson of the HMOs in the United States is that they provide a mechanism for achieving the most cost-effective use of medical resources in the interests of their members, providing them with better standards of health and, when they need it, of medical treatment. They offer a model well worthy of study, and in my view of emulation, in this country. In Chapter Ten I set out some ideas on how HMOs might be adapted to solve our problems.

During the last few years the concept of the Preferred Provider Organisation (PPO) has emerged in the United States as an alternative method of paying for medical treatment, offering a half-way house between the traditional fee-for-services arrangement and the HMO. A feature of the HMO system is that it locks the subscriber paying his monthly premium firmly into the organi-sation so that if, for example, he decides to consult a specialist who is not on the HMO panel he would have no insurance cover.

PPOs contract with selected hospitals and doctors to offer services to insurers and purchasers (employers) at negotiated prices, which may be up to 30 or even 40% less than the prevailing rate. The arrangement is attractive to both hospitals and doctors as they are paid directly by the insurer, thus avoiding the need for individual billing and the risk of bad debts, and it gives them the opportunity to increase their market share. The subscriber benefits from the lower charges from the PPO doctors, is protected from inadequate treatment by internal utilisation review procedures and still enjoys insurance cover (even though possibly without 100% reimbursement) should he decide to use an outside hospital or specialist.

The principle of negotiated rates for identified groups was, in fact, the basis of the Blue Cross and Blue Shield Plans in the 1930s and '40s but the PPO phenomenon is a much more recent growth as insurers and employers have looked for new ways of keeping medical costs under control. A survey reported that there were 33 PPOs in 1982. By 1985 there were 325, with 5.5 million subscribers enrolled.

The explosion in American medical costs is now generating changes in the providers and the services they offer. In the face of growing resistance from the consumers and the payers — the government and local authorities, the insurers and the employers — hospitals and doctors have begun to look to ways of delivering adequate health care more economically. This is why many are now co-operating in, and often promoting, PPOs.

Another innovation by American providers which would repay examination as a possible way of improving medical services in the United Kingdom is the development of free-standing ambulatory surgical centres. These travelling centres, some organised by hospitals and others by independent groups of doctors, offer a limited range of surgical procedures that can be performed safely and successfully outside the hospital, thus saving the insurer and the patient all the costs and inconvenience of hospitalisation. They were an instant success when first introduced and have now been followed by the creation of "emergicentres", primary care centres, diagnostic centres and others.

I thought it right to dwell at some length on the American experience as it provides many examples, both bad (which we hear about) and good (which we don't), which could be useful in our search for better health services in Britain. There can be no doubt or challenge that the best of American medicine is very good indeed and that over wide areas they have achieved standards which we could not hope to match in this country under our present system. It also seems — these are relatively early days — that many of their efforts to contain costs are taking effect, whilst the general health of the American people continues to improve.

One great advantage they have over us is that most Americans see health care as a national issue involving the whole of society; they have not been conditioned by forty years of the NHS to regard it as almost exclusively a *government* responsibility and simply a matter of extracting more money out of the Chancellor of the Exchequer. A manifestation of this attitude is seen in the emergence of "health coalitions" throughout the United States in which employers, trade unions, insurers, the providers of health services, local authorities and other bodies all join to find ways of reducing medical costs and to promote health and fitness prog-rammes in their communities.

Health promotion and preventive medicine is another area where we compare badly with the United States. The "managed care" approach discussed earlier involves a positive approach to health which is almost completely absent from the NHS system, a deficiency which was pointed out at the time of its creation and has not been made good since. American insurers and employers strongly encourage subscribers to look after themselves. There are discounts for non-smokers and many "wellness" programmes which offer keep-fit facilities, health education and regular monitoring of conditions such as high blood pressure.

The results are coming through in the whole range of medical statistics used to make international comparisons of performance. One important indicator, for example, is the trend in the rate of deaths from coronary heart disease and the American record of achievement in this area has been very impressive in recent years. In 1971, taking the standard WHO figures for death rates per 100,000 males between the ages of 35 and 74, American men had one of the highest in the world at 743, compared with a figure for England and Wales of 592. By 1980 the Americans had brought their rate down to 491, a reduction of 34%. During the same period we had made virtually no improvement, recording a figure of 587. American women did even better, achieving a reduction of nearly 38%. The figure for England and Wales actually increased slightly, from 197 in 1971 to 199 in 1980.

Statistics like these graphically demonstrate the effectiveness of the sort of "wellness" programmes which have been generated by the American experience and the dismal failure of the NHS in the area of preventive medicine. And, of course, these are not just statistics in a political and economic debate; we are talking about many thousands of people who are suffering and dying prematurely because of our failure to adopt a more sensible system of health care.

As we consider how we can make better provision for our health services in Britain, we should certainly remember that the Americans have been spending about 11% of a GNP which, per capita, is very much higher than ours and the plight of the uninsured 10% who must have recourse to low-grade public hospitals when they are sick. But we should also take account of what the Americans have achieved and, in particular, what they have learned in recent years.

Lessons from the Rest of the World

The great diversity of health care systems limits the value of comparisons and of the lessons which can be drawn from the experience of other countries. Nevertheless, certain broad trends serve at least to offer pointers to the way we should reform the British system.

Our starting point always has to be that, with the (now changing) exception of New Zealand, no other country has adopted a system modelled on what we were pleased to call "the envy of the world"; one or two flirted briefly with some of the basic principles of the NHS but tip-toed away again. We should therefore at least recognise the possibility that other advanced democracies may have something to teach us.

We have already noted (Chapter Seven) that the pressures creating increased health spending have caused it to absorb a rising proportion of the national wealth in every country — with the proportion rising more slowly in Britain than in many others. During the late 1960s and the 1970s, in particular, this phenomenon was accompanied by a tendency in all countries for the publicly-financed share of this spending to grow, the OECD average increasing from 61% in 1960 to 76% in 1975.[3] We have seen above that this even happened in the United States, especially after 1965.

This trend had levelled out by 1980 and is now being put into reverse, as governments become increasingly determined to check increases in public spending and to keep health costs under control. In Australia, for example, Gough Whitlam's Labour Government introduced the Medibank scheme in 1975 which took the public proportion of health spending up from 64 to 75%. The present Labour government is now changing the system, which already demands far more from the individual than does the NHS, and proposes to shift more of the funding burden back to the private sector. The Medicare scheme introduced in Australia in 1984 provided only 85% of medical fees, on a fixed national scale, and free treatment only in public hospitals and without choice of doctor. The introduction of Medicare produced higher expenditure, long hospital waiting lists, disruption and a strike in the most populous state, New South Wales, which threatened to close many public hospitals. The Government was thrown into hasty retreat and by 1st September 1985 was obliged to introduce further changes aimed at increasing the number of private patients and expanding the private sector.

In the Netherlands, too, a substantial rise in recent years in the health costs carried by the Government is now leading to a switch to more insurance in the private sector. In 1974, when the Dutch were riding high on the benefits of their North Sea earnings, central government began to play a larger role in the funding and organisation of health care. A two-tier system was created under which roughly two-thirds of the population were covered by government insurance and the more affluent third by private insurance. A separate Government fund covered the whole population against expenses not provided for by either insurance system. The public insurance scheme was funded by a percentage of income fixed every year and paid equally by employee and employer (4.8% from each). Premiums for the private insurance schemes varied according to the level of benefits.

The public insurance scheme led to overly expensive or unnecessary treatment and more in-patient and less out-patient treatment in hospitals, with a consequent rise in costs. By 1986 the Dutch were spending 8.5% of their Gross National Product, or the equivalent of £564 per head, on their health services. The Netherlands Government is now again reducing its involvement in the health field and "partial reforms" were introduced in April 1986, following which 750,000 people formerly in the public scheme took out private insurance.

There are quite close parallels with the situation in West Germany. Those earning under about £18,000 a year (1987) are covered by a government insurance scheme, with employees and employers both paying 6% of gross earnings into the fund. Revenue for public sector health spending is also obtained from Federal, State and local taxation, direct charges and co-payments made by consumers and additional charges on employers (who pay a sickness allowance of up to six weeks). German health spending increased from 8.9% of GNP in 1980 to 9.2% in 1985 (the equivalent of £722 per head) and concern at this rate of growth has led to a re-examination of the system. It is now recognised that complete insurance coverage creates the "moral hazard" of the consumer placing unlimited and unreasonable demands on the system, often encouraged by the doctors (who in Germany earn five times the average wage compared with two and a half times in Britain). Proposals are therefore in hand to increase the arrangements for co-payments and to introduce others by means of improving the level of cost-consciousness in both patients and providers.

Canada's health care arrangements are based on a mix of the three systems of funding considered by British politicians and administrators in the '30s and '40s, national, regional and insurance — the first of which being selected by Bevan for the NHS. The provinces run medical insurance programmes which must satisfy criteria established by the federal government. Provinces are responsible for the delivery of the health care services but about 40% of their spending, on a *per capita* basis, is met by grants from the national government. Out of total health spending about a quarter comes directly out of the pocket of the individual or his insurer and it seems likely that this proportion will grow in the future. *Per capita* health spending grew at a compound rate of over 10% between 1970 and 1984 to US $1,275 or 9.2% of GDP. Converting in terms of purchasing power parity, this was over twice the level of spending in Britain. Not surprisingly, the Canadians are now anxiously studying the cost-containing experience of their southern neighbours.

The country regarded by many as having a health system which is closest to the socialist model of the NHS is Sweden. It is true that it is second only to Britain in the proportion of health spending which is funded out of general taxation but the crucial difference is that some 95% of that funding in Sweden is raised on a county rather than a national basis. It is thus on the lines of the scheme favoured by the Labour Party Congress and, as late as 1946, by Herbert Morrison but which was successfully resisted by Aneurin Bevan. The difficulties we have had in finding a satisfactory method of financing local government and the failure of several attempts to create autonomous health regions noted in Chapter Five, demonstrate that, even if it offered other advantages, the Swedish model could not be translated to this country.

Virtually all other advanced countries have adopted some form of insurance scheme to fund their health care, with a varying degree of government involvement; none has opted for anything like the NHS system. To put it in British terms, they have chosen to go along the Lloyd George route rather than take the diversion down which Aneurin Bevan led us after the Second World War.

Insurance schemes have demonstrated they are more flexible, and thus better able to cope with changing and increasing demands, and are more open-ended, and thus much better at promoting private health spending. It is therefore not surprising to find that, by whichever method the calculations are made, spending on health in other industrialised countries tends to be between 50% and 100% greater than in Britain — and in some, much more.

But it is easy to agree that the level of spending is not the criterion which, in the end, matters. It is therefore also important to note that, with all their problems, the systems in other countries have within them greater incentives to efficiency than we have here. Consequently, the level of health care enjoyed by the citizens of many other countries is, in general, better than that available to the British. They have no experience, for example, of the sort of waiting times for hospital admission that we have accepted for decades.

Other countries have also found another advantage over us in their arrangements for health care. Whilst it is an issue which is, inevitably, a matter of political debate and economic judgement, they have managed to keep it far from the level of political controversy which has become such a distinctive feature of the

NHS, for which nearly all the funding comes directly from the national exchequer.

No country would claim to have solved the health dilemma and I have outlined above some of the problems they face. They will always need to fight to keep the pressures and the costs under control and increase the awareness of all involved about the realities of finite resources. Thus there is likely to be an extension of the "co-payment" approach, perhaps along the lines of the "ticket moderateur" which has operated in France and Belgium for years — under which most patients themselves pay for their treatment in the first instance and are able only to recover about three-quarters from the fund.

So we all have problems to solve — but Britain has more than most. American and West European experience offers us many lessons; some of them negative, some very positive. The essential thing now is that we must learn from them without more delay.

9

Some Roads Worth Exploring

The effectiveness of the National Health Service or any reform or replacement of it must be judged against a set of criteria very different from those accepted just after the Second World War. It should:

* promote an increase in health spending of about 50% — to put Britain on a par with other advanced European countries. In 1988 terms this means something of the order of £10-11,000 million.

* generate this money from sources other than the national Exchequer — otherwise there would be a catastrophic effect on the economy and no remedy of the structural weaknesses of the NHS.

* take account of the fact that British society is now much changed, is far more affluent and needs a very different health service from what seemed adequate in 1946. The NHS was planned to deal with acute disease rather than to deliver modern health care or "wellness".

* embody controls which will ensure that the enhanced budget (which will certainly still leave some demands unmet) is properly used. This will require changes in the work style of many doctors and other providers, who have taken advantage

of the weaknesses of the NHS structure to avoid the discip-
lines that are essential if expensive medical resources are to be
used to best effect.

* provide a comprehensive service so that good *managed* health
care is available to all — a much more positive concept than
the NHS has been able to offer.

* create for the British consumer the sort of choice that a citizen
of a modern and prosperous country has a right to expect.

If we accept these criteria, fundamental changes in our present
arrangements are inescapable. None of the devices for making the
same amount of money go further, some of which we considered in
Chapter Six — an "internal market" in the NHS, better management, competitive tendering, fund raising activities or "hotel
charges" by hospitals — would be capable of providing the answer.
And without fundamental change of the NHS structure we shall
still have the organisational weaknesses which have survived forty
years of attempts at reform and have been a constant source of
political tension without producing an acceptable standard of
management of the individual's health needs.

Some people, too terrorised by the political power of the NHS
myth to propose or even support radical change, cling to the hope
that salvation will be found in the natural growth of private medical
insurance. This view, which we have already considered briefly
(Chapter 6, page 95), is held by members of most political
parties and certainly by some members of the Conservative
Government — who are regularly and very unjustifiably accused of
deliberately starving the NHS of resources precisely in order to
stimulate a switch to private medicine.

There can be no hope in merely waiting for growth in the private
insurance sector to relieve the pressures on the NHS. The number
of subscribers to private medical insurance doubled in the decade
from 1975 but the rate of increase declined thereafter. About 10%
of the population now have some form of private cover, the great
majority through company schemes. Private spending on health

accounts for only a small proportion of the total (about 6%) and unless there is some extraordinary change in present trends, there is no prospect in the foreseeable future that, within the existing structure, the private sector can rescue the NHS from its agonies.

One school of thought maintains that growth in the private sector could be stimulated to the point where it makes a significant contribution by granting tax incentives to insurance schemes and their subscribers. I believe this proposition is highly questionable and would certainly run into many difficulties. It would be costly to the Exchequer and would go against the present and entirely sensible taxation policy which aims to reduce the number of tax allowances rather than increase them. In itself it would do nothing to improve or eliminate the weaknesses we have noted in the NHS. Most importantly of all in political terms it would lead to emotive charges of "two-tier" treatment, two nations and all the rest which would be very damaging — despite the fact that opinion polls show a significant degree of support for the idea. It would probably result in the government of the day *increasing* spending on the NHS in an attempt to rebut such allegations.

There would be still other pitfalls in an attempt to find an insurance solution to the health dilemma. The growth in private tax allowances would be seen as exacerbating further the North-South divide. In fact, as it operates at present medical insurance has had only a very limited effect on the demand for NHS facilities. It provides little or no cover for general practice or emergency care or for long-term treatment of chronic conditions such as mental illness. The bulk of spending by the insurers is for about thirty categories of non-emergency ("cold") surgery — "running repairs" such as hernias, varicose veins, haemorrhoids and minor gynaecological procedures (which explains why among the medical profession, private medicine is defended very much more vigorously by surgeons than by physicians).

Another approach to the problem which has been gaining ground in recent years goes like this: "whilst lower taxes are, for obvious reasons, popular and sensible in broader economic terms, people understand the need and would be ready to pay more for adequate

health services — provided only that the tax system clearly identified that the payments they made went directly and exclusively to
the NHS."

Such a solution would, of course, do nothing to cure many of the
weaknesses of the NHS we have identified and could well make
some of them worse. The pressures to contain costs would be eased
and there would be no incentive to provide managed health care
tailored to the needs of the individual. Even with a 50% increase in
resources, many demands would go unmet so there would still be
political tensions.

These drawbacks are serious enough — but the financial effects
of such a strategy would be even worse. If we considered the
proposition in terms of 1987-8 spending, the 50% increase in health
spending that we have accepted as being "needed" to bring us up to
international levels, would amount to some £10 billion. Let us
assume that it was decided that we would change the arrangements
for the National Insurance Fund, to which employees and employers pay their National Insurance Contributions (NIC's). At
present most of this Fund is committed to the payment of social
security benefits and it provides for only 13% of NHS expenditure.
It would be possible to use the NIC's as the exclusive and sole
source of NHS money, thus creating a special fund which, for
convenience, we might call here the Dedicated Health Fund. The
DHF would be insulated from income tax and the general Exchequer system and many believe that there would be a ready
acceptance of the concept, given the depth of public support for the
NHS and the importance attached to good health care.

The consequence of a change on these lines would, however, be
wide-ranging and serious. To accommodate the 50% increase in the
NHS budget we are seeking it would be necessary to raise the NIC
rate for employees from 9% to 10% (preserving the 5 and 7% rates
for those on low incomes and an upper limit of £305 per week) and
that of employers from the present 10.45% to 11.75%.

These figures allow for the preservation of the existing arrangement under which companies with their own pension schemes are
allowed to "contract out" and pay reduced NIC rates — 2% less for

the employee and 4% less for the employer. This would mean that those in the State Earnings Related Pensions Scheme would be carrying a heavier share of the health burden — but to abolish the rebate would be a mortal blow to occupational pension schemes.

But the concept of a DHF has other, and still more worrying, drawbacks. In order to fund from general taxation the social security budget which is at present met from the National Insurance Fund, it would be necessary to increase the basic rate of income tax by no less than 5p in the pound!

The effect of the DHF is probably seen most graphically in its impact on staff actually working in the NHS. *It would mean that the deductions from the salary of a nursing sister earning £12,000 a year would be increased by nearly £14 a week.* This is a figure that those advocating a solution on these lines, which would leave unresolved the other problems of the NHS, should ponder.

Some of the staunchest defenders of the NHS, who argue that the service needs a massive injection of funds, claim that this could be found from swingeing extra taxes either on tobacco products alone or on tobacco and alcohol. They support their case by referring to the extra burdens on the NHS which result from smoking and excessive use of alcohol.

The briefest look at the figures, however, demonstrates the impracticality of these ideas. In order to raise the £10 billion which would bring health spending in Britain at least roughly into line with other West European countries it would be necessary to increase the duty on cigarettes to the point where a packet of 20 would cost £4! The impact of such an increase is easy to imagine.

Spreading the burden to include alcohol would produce a result only marginally less acceptable. For example, the money could be found — subject to the crucial caveat that consumption was not deterred — by *increasing* existing duty (January 1988) by 87p on a pint of beer, £1.50 on a bottle of wine, £2.50 on a bottle of spirits and 90p on a packet of cigarettes.

It has also become fashionable to say that all that is required is for the Government to accept that the pressures for increased health spending (that terrible trio I will not repeat yet again) can be catered for by providing for a growth in the NHS budget of 2% in real terms every year. 2% does not sound much but the cumulative effect would be disastrous.

Given that the total of public spending was held steady in real terms, a 2% increase for the NHS would mean that the 13% of expenditure it accounted for in 1987-88 would rise to 21.3% in twenty-five years. This would involve massive misery spread across the rest of the public sector or, for example, the elimination of *all* spending on transport, housing, overseas aid and arts and libraries.

Another possible option would be for the Government to establish a tariff of fees for treatment, on the lines of the diagnosis related groups developed in the United States and discussed in Chapters Six and Eight. These fees could be paid at the standard rate to whoever provided the service, whether in or outside the NHS. A variation would be to retain present arrangements for the NHS but pay a fixed proportion, say 65%, of costs incurred by a patient in the private sector.

Such a system would involve the Government in an annual task of setting the rates. This would be a fruitful area of contention, as the experience of countries such as Australia and Belgium have demonstrated. An added complication in Britain would arise from the fact that costing procedures in the NHS itself are still lamentably underdeveloped. There would probably need to be regional differences in rates — another source of trouble — and if certain fee services became manifestly more profitable than others the result could be a wasteful misallocation of resources. It is a system that would be best suited to hospital care. There would be difficulties with primary and long-term care and in creating proper incentives to avoid waste and misuse. It could end up as an arrangement that made the Common Agricultural Policy look simple and sensible by comparison.

There is another range of possible solutions which would depend on establishing clear NHS costings for every treatment, stay in hospital etc. and then presenting the patient with the bill, in the manner of the *ticket moderateur* in France and Belgium. Special categories (the elderly, the chronic sick and those below an established income level) would be totally exempt from paying towards the cost. Other patients would be responsible for paying a proportion, which could be a fixed percentage — say 15% — or a fixed sum up to a set limit — say up to the first £50 — or might be recovered on annual basis through the income tax mechanism so that payment would be related to income, with an upper limit to help those who incur expensive treatment.

Any arrangement on these lines would have the benefit of introducing a perception of costs to both patients and providers which is notably absent from the NHS at present. It would also, however, have obvious drawbacks. It would be necessary to create a whole new administrative structure to handle the accounting requirements, with the NHS billing itself and then, for the most part, paying itself. It would leave intact the administrative structure of the NHS, with most of its weaknesses unaffected. In itself, such a scheme would not introduce any additional funding into health care and there would, again, be problems for the government in setting rates which would be accepted as fair by providers throughout the country and yet not cripplingly high. In political terms it is a very unattractive option.

With the growing realisation that the gap will continue to widen between public expectations and the capacity of the NHS, as currently organised and funded, to deliver, one solution increasingly advocated is the launch of a national lottery to supplement health care resources. I certainly have no objection in principle to gambling or lotteries but I have to confess to an instinctive distaste of the proposition that something as important as the nation's health should depend on the proceeds of a lottery. I believe very many people would have the same reaction.

In any case, the evidence available does not suggest that a lottery would be likely to generate the sort of funds needed to bring our health services up to the standards we want. The Peacock Committee, considering the future of the BBC in 1985, also looked into the possibility of using lotteries as a source of funding and produced some interesting findings. They looked at four countries where lotteries are used extensively to generate revenue for the public sector or for charitable causes — West Germany, Spain, France and the United States. They found that in Germany the weekly State Lottery in 1983 produced about £700 million for these purposes. The National Lottery in Spain produced some £500 million in 1982 and the three main lotteries in France a total of about £550 million in 1984. There is no national lottery system in the USA but there are lotteries in many States and the Peacock figures suggest that taken together they generate something over £1 billion annually. A feature of the lotteries was what Peacock described as the "amazingly high" per capita sales by the lotteries in each country — £21 a year in France, £29 in Germany, £45 in Spain and £99 in the State of New Jersey. All the evidence suggests that, even were a health service lottery to become firmly established in Britain — a process which would surely take years — the most it would be likely to produce would be about £500 million. The fact is that we already have a national lottery which is much more deeply rooted here than in any other country — the football pools — and it is difficult to imagine that they will ever be displaced.

A variation of this idea is the proposal that the principle of the premium bonds lottery should be adapted to provide additional funds for the NHS. Again, all experience suggests that such a scheme would have no chance at all for generating the sort of money that is needed. At present premium bonds produce about £80 million a year. And like the other possible remedies for the health care dilemma discussed above, lotteries and premium bonds would leave untouched many of the basic failings of the NHS — and might even make them worse. Given the additional source of funding, the medical and nursing professions would certainly step up their pressure for more resources and higher pay, together with their resistance to attempts to get them to accept costing and budgetting procedures which were long ago adopted by their counterparts in other countries.

Yet another suggestion — a lot of effort is being expended to avoid the political challenge involved in facing up to the real need to reform the NHS! — is that all would be well if we instituted just one more structural change. It will be recalled that in 1982 the Conservative Government abolished the Area Health Authorities as a tier of administration (Chapter Five, page 75). A more recent proposal is that the Regional Health Authorities should be abolished.

As I can certainly attest from personal experience, Health Ministers and the DHSS already find it difficult enough to deal with the 14 Regional Authorities. Should the RHA's be dismantled, they would then be required to handle 192 District Health Authorities. The financial, organisational and political tensions would be very much worse even than they are at present. Whereas it is possible to maintain a level of group loyalty between the 14 Regional Chairmen and the Health Ministers, this would be out of the question with a much larger number. Instead, there would develop a fierce and very public competition among the 192 Chairmen with each trying to shout the loudest to get more funds for his district. And, again, the likely savings would come nowhere near to meeting the needs of the NHS. The administrative costs of *both* tiers of health authority, region and district, in England in 1985-86 amounted to only £374 million.

A much more promising suggestion is that the NHS should adopt the concept of Health Maintenance Organisations, benefitting from the American experience. One version of this, proposed by Dr Eamonn Butler, is that groups of NHS general practitioners should be invited or encouraged to set up their own HMO's, receiving a premium for each NHS patient they are able to attract. He has suggested that, following the lines of the Medicare scheme in the United States, the DHSS should assess the average cost of each individual dependent on the NHS and pay that sum as an annual premium to the group practice. He believes it might even be slightly less, like the Medicare arrangement, in recognition of the greater cost-efficiency the system is likely to produce. The setting of the premiums would clearly be a difficult aspect of the arrangement. They would presumably have to vary with the age or medical history of the patients; otherwise the HMO would accept only the relatively healthy or consider itself aggrieved if obliged by the system to accept a proportion of potentially more costly patients without adequate recompense.

Once the premium is paid, the HMO would be under contract to provide all necessary treatment (another problem area). This would, of course, require them to contract with specialists and hospitals, either in the private sector or the NHS. In the case of the latter, it would be necessary to establish a reasonable and realistic scale of charges for the treatment that would be provided. Butler takes comfort from the findings of a Rand Corporation study of the American experience, which showed that HMO's, in addition to producing a clear improvement in patient satisfaction, tended to reduce hospitalisation by 40%. The consequent reduction in the notorious hospital waiting lists would be very welcome to the government of the day.

Butler also suggests that a one-off grant might be made to groups of general practitioners prepared to establish a Health Maintenance Organisation. This would enable them to equip their surgeries to provide more facilities for testing, diagnosis and minor surgery in order to reduce the recourse to hospitals for either in- or out-patient treatment. Patients would much prefer treatment by their own local doctors whenever possible, both because the relationship is more personal and in order to avoid the disturbance, travel and long waiting involved in hospital treatment.

I believe there are many attractions in the HMO system, which at its best provides the consumer with the advantages of choice and a higher level of managed care than the NHS can offer, whilst keeping costs under control. One interesting and important experiment in establishing the concept in this country was launched by the Harrow Health Centre in 1982, under the energetic leadership of Dr Michael Goldsmith. For £140 a year it provided full primary care, drugs and out-patient hospital treatment, which could be complemented by hospital cover from Private Patients Plan at a basic premium of £150 a year. The Centre has now switched to a fee-for-service arrangement because, set firmly within the ambience of the NHS, it was dealing with individuals whereas the HMO idea needs the group approach to be really successful and effective. It is, however, still going strong.

I am very doubtful whether HMO's could be introduced into this country on a satisfactory basis without much more significant changes in the NHS than Dr Butler had in mind. General practitioners are too comfortably ensconced in the existing arrangements, which happily combine for them the security of the health service with the benefits of the status of "independent contractor". Other reforms would be needed before many (or even any) could be persuaded to take on the financial risks and administrative burdens which HMO's would involve. Whilst doctors are as attracted by material rewards as the rest of us — indeed one of them told me that "the only way to deliver a message to a doctor is to write it on a cheque" — forty years of the NHS has withered the entrepreneurial spirit.

I believe there *is* a way to bring about those other reforms which will be needed if HMO's are to take root and flourish and I offer my ideas on how that might be achieved in the next chapter, where I set out my own solution to the health conundrum.

10
A Modern Solution to an Old Problem

The major objective of this book is to carry forward the debate on health provision in Britain which is so long overdue but which has now begun.

In this Chapter I offer the outline of my own solution to the NHS conundrum which, I believe, could provide us with a health service which would be modern, comprehensive and sensitive to the needs of the individual — the sort of health service we have a right to expect in a caring and affluent society. It is based on my experience as a DHSS Minister and the daily contact with the welfare services which is normal for a Member of Parliament, together with what I have learned from studying the efforts made in Britain and in many other countries over several decades to find answers to the same problems.

It is an outline which would need much more detailed work before it could be implemented — and which will certainly be fiercely criticised by those who hope they will be able to preserve the *status quo* merely by demanding yet more Treasury money or by waving a fig-leaf of manifestly superficial reforms. I believe, however, that the proposals I set out below offer the framework for a new system of health care which could combine the best of British and foreign experience.

As we saw in earlier chapters, our predecessors since at least 1911 recognised that, in essence, there were three methods of delivering health care — on an insurance basis, through a regional or local structure or by an organisation centrally controlled and funded. Faced with the same options, virtually every other democratic industrialised country chose either an insurance or a regionally organised system, although of course each one ended up with a distinctive recipe — or series of recipes — of its own.

In Britain we had been one of the first in the field with an insurance system and by 1945 about half the population (those with incomes under £420 a year) were covered by Lloyd George's scheme. It would have been possible to develop and extend that arrangement in the manner which has since proved effective in other countries, who now enjoy better health services than we do, with much less political bitterness and a smaller drain on their national exchequer. After forty years of painful experience it should be clear to all but the most purblind that Bevan made a grave mistake in taking us off the insurance path and that we should now get back on to it.

By the end of the war there was a strong tide running for the idea that medical services should be organised on a local basis. Many — including Bevan (see Chapter 3, page 34) — saw the dangers of a system controlled by a centralised bureaucracy and it was widely believed that a locally-based organisation would be much more sensitive to the needs of the community and of the individual. As I recorded in Chapter Three, the Labour Party Conference in 1944 voted for the transfer of hospitals and medical services to local authorities and in February 1946 Herbert Morrison was still saying that "the view of the Minister of Health and the Government was that it would not be right to take the hospitals over into a national concern". Within a few weeks the Minister of Health, Bevan, had defeated him in the Cabinet battle and had carried the nation into the centralised structure that, ever since, we have been trying to operate. The scheme I outline in this chapter offers another opportunity to create hospitals and other services which would be based on and controlled by the local community, free at last of the national bureaucracy to which Herbert Morrison and his Labour colleagues justifiably objected.

In our search for an improved system of health care there are two points which need to be borne in mind but which I have so far given little emphasis. The first is that there is no absolute requirement for the system of *paying* for health care and the arrangements for *delivering* that care to be directly linked in the way they are in the NHS. Indeed, as we have seen, in those countries where the two functions are separated a better result is usually produced. This outcome is entirely to be expected because when the responsibility for both paying and providing rests ultimately in the same hands there is no incentive to set up the costing mechanisms which seem natural in many other forms of human activity and enable us to make sensible judgements about the best use of limited resources. We thus suffer the paradox that whilst there is a keen appreciation that there is a *general* pressure on NHS funds those working within the service have, to a damaging extent, been able to resist the introduction of sensible measures of budgetary measurement and control in the treatment of cases, where it is much needed.

It is precisely because of the absence of costing data in the NHS that is is very difficult to make detailed comparisons with costs in the private sector or in other countries. However, I can offer one example given to me by Mr John Hughes, who was Chairman of a private company, Community Dialysis Services. The Welsh Health Authority decided to put the provision of dialysis facilities out to private tender and Community Dialysis Services was one of the companies awarded a contract. CDS were able to provide the service at a charge of £78 per treatment in 1986-87. This price included the cost of capital, depreciation, interest and the company's profit. Given the absence of proper cost-control data in the NHS, CDS ran into problems when they tried to get comparative figures from the 14 Regional Health Authorities. Eventually Yorkshre RHA — to their credit — were able to produce figures from which it was possible to make a reasonable estimate of the cost of "in centre" hospital dialysis. This worked out at £143.49 per treatment. The two figures are not strictly comparable as Yorkshire's figures *presumably* include an element for medical staff expenditure, which is not in the CDS costing. On the other hand, the NHS figures contain no allowance for capital charges etc. and therefore the comparison is almost certainly not far off target. The estimate of the North East Thames Regional Health Authority for the cost of dialysis treatment in 1986 was "somewhere between £120 and £150" — a very wide bracket given that every year many thousands of treatments are performed.

The second point to be remembered might be summarised in the cliché about the best being the enemy of the good. For over a generation it was a matter of clear agreement between all British political parties that the health service should provide *equal* access to the *best* care for everyone and that this service should be without regard to cost. As we saw in the 1944 White Paper produced by the Conservative Health Minister, the objective was that "in future every man, woman and child can rely on getting all the advice and treatment and care which they may need in matters of personal health; that what they get shall be the best medical and other facilities available."

Inevitably, this objective was adopted by Aneurin Bevan when he launched the NHS and over the years has become the regular stand-by of any Labour politician making a speech on health. It is, for example, the sort of concept that fits in very well with the emotional but unthinking approach of Mr Neil Kinnock. Equally inevitably, however, it has always proved to be an objective that was unrealistic and unattainable. In providing medical care it will never be possible — and sometimes may not even be sensible to try — to ensure that everyone is given the best service. After twenty years experience of the NHS the force of that logic was accepted by the Labour Health Minister of the day, Kenneth Robinson, and in his foreword to his 1968 Green Paper he redefined the aims of the NHS in much more balanced terms, as follows:

> The paramount requirement is that all the different kinds of care and treatment that an individual may need at different times, whether separately or in combination, should be readily available to him.

That is the criterion by which any reform or replacement of the

NHS should be judged and which would be met by the scheme I propose below.

In large measure it is based on the work and the conclusions of an Advisory Planning Panel commissioned by the British Medical Association in 1967 under the chairmanship of a Hertfordshire general practitioner, Dr Ivor Jones. Early that year the then Chairman of Council of the BMA, Dr Ronald Gibson, invited Jones to set up a committee "to undertake research and enquiry into the National Health Service from its origins and indicate possible trends for the future."

Such was the state of anxiety among the medical profession about the condition and the prospects of the NHS at the time, however, that in July 1967 the Representative Body of the BMA adopted a resolution which gave Dr Jones a much more challenging remit and called for the urgent preparation of an alternative health service in which financial provision would be less dependent on taxation. It is a bitterly ironic commentary that after twenty more years of the NHS, when there is general agreement that the service is under very much greater pressure, when there is a great deal more evidence that the Bevan formula does not work and when British society has demonstrated since 1979 how well it can respond to change, it would be unthinkable to hope that the modern BMA would pass a resolution imbued with a similar level of radical open-mindedness.

Ten of the twelve members of the Jones panel were from the medical profession — four GP's, five consultants and one County Medical Officer. One of the lay members was the economist, Mr Arthur Seldon, whose insights show through clearly in the final report. The other was a young Barrister at Law with political aspirations, Mr Geoffrey Howe, QC.

The committee worked for two years and published its findings in April 1970. Its report of the shortcomings of the NHS might have been written at any time since ... "performance ... is shown to compare unfavourably with that of many other countries in several respects" ... "inadequate finance both in regard to capital running costs." ... "the imperfections of our health service are clearly visible" ..."staffing is deficient at all levels and many sections are underpaid" ... "it appears probable that Britain must think in terms of additional expenditure on medical care of an order which no Government has ever contemplated". It all has a very contemporary ring.

The essence of the Jones' proposals was that Britain should revert to an insurance system, whilst reserving certain services to be centrally funded from taxation. The committee recommended that everyone should be entitled to "compulsory health insurance", the premiums for which would be deducted from individual incomes through the Inland Revenue but paid into an entirely separate fund. People could contract out of this arrangement if they joined "voluntary health insurance" schemes which offered higher benefits through the payment of higher premiums. The report suggested that the lowest income groups should pay little or nothing for compulsory insurance cover, the premium increasing gradually until those earning the national average income (about £1,000 in 1968) would pay the full rate.

It was assumed that people earning above that level would start opting for voluntary health insurance and the Jones committee saw this as the source of the new funds which the NHS needed so badly. They firmly refused to make any attempt to "quantify precisely the additional money required to raise the standard of medical care to an acceptable level" but suggested that there were "cogent reasons" for believing that the sum required was "substantially in excess" of £500 million a year. The imprecision is clearly deliberate but they seem to have had in mind an increase in national (not government) spending on health care of around 40%. It is not surprising that over twenty years later we appear likely to need a little more than that. The Jones committee believed that the experience of other countries demonstrated that people were willing to devote more of their personal resources to their own medical care once they were involved in a system which made them aware of the link between money and the cost and quality of the services they received. They pointed out that at the time the nation was spending £25,000 million on other goods and services and that a "switch of only a small percentage of this annual expenditure to the health services would achieve all that is necessary."

The force of that logic is even stronger in a country which, twenty years on, is much richer. In 1986 the total household *disposable* income (that is after payment of income taxes and NIC's) was £244,000 million — a figure which, in cash terms, more than trebled in a decade. £10,000 million diverted to health spending would involve only some 4% of disposable income, which is surely a very modest figure for something as important as health care.

There were two areas in which the Jones committee were more cautious than we can now afford — or need — to be. They were very conscious "of the disadvantages so apparent in the current American system", pointing to the inflationary impact on health costs of the insurance approach, the limitations imposed on benefits, the foreclosure on "bad risks" and so on. In part, at least, as a response to these concerns they opted for what would, I believe, have become a cumbersome hybrid and opted for the creation of two distinct insurance sectors, the "compulsory" and the "voluntary".

This is something we can now avoid, by taking advantage of two more decades of experience in many countries, but particularly in the United States, in devising techniques which ensure that the highly beneficial effects of the insurance system are retained and developed whilst the potentially inflationary effects are kept under control. We can now devise one insurance structure to cover the nation. There are often advantages in arriving late.

The other area where the Jones committee demonstrated caution was in its approach to the NHS itself. They concluded that "it is neither desirable nor practicable to think in terms of dismantling of the NHS", suggesting that it would be "more constructive and realistic" to propose "an administrative structure which will make possible the most efficient use of all resources available for health services in Britain, without compromising the essential freedoms of both the professions and the public." In reaching this conclusion Dr Jones and his colleagues reflected the conservative (small "c") attitudes of the majority of the medical profession, the aura with which the NHS had become surrounded and the optimism that just a few more changes in structure, backed up by a massive injection of new funds, would solve the administrative problems of the NHS. After twenty more years of administrative changes and a huge rise in government spending there can be no surviving grounds for such optimism.

Regrettably, in both the interests of the nation as a whole and of the NHS itself, when it appeared in April 1970 the Jones report fell on ground which had turned to stone. By then the Government had ended its dispute with the doctors on terms the profession thought acceptable and the medico-political climate had changed. The BMA therefore cold-shouldered the report it had itself commissioned and Britain's system of health care continued on the path which has led us directly to today's problems. Dr Ivor Jones, who was, in the words of his obituary in the *British Medical Journal* in 1987, "arguably the most dominant figure in medico-politics in the 1960's", was abruptly dropped by the medical establishment. Having played a leading role in negotiating the *GP Charter* with the Government, he was the only one of the BMA negotiators whose name did not subsequently appear in the Honours Lists. As the *BMJ* observed nearly twenty years later, "those who succeed through proving that the established point of view is flawed rarely receive the honours that are due to them".[1]

A Modern Solution

I believe we should now move to a system which is based on the *funding* of health care by the allocation of vouchers or credits to the individual and the *provision* of services through health maintenance organisations or insurance-supported alternatives and, at the secondary level, autonomous hospitals. The operation of the system would be monitored and controlled by a National Health Authority. We should be building on the ideas of Lloyd George and Herbert Morrison and escaping from Aneurin Bevan's cul-de-sac.

Each individual would be entitled to a health credit or voucher, provided by the Government. They would then be required to arrange satisfactory medical cover with an authorised provider of primary care, who would then accept responsibility for the delivery of any hospital and specialist treatment which might be needed. General practitioners would be expected, where necessary, to assist all those on their lists to complete the necessary formalities, in order to ensure that no-one "fell through the net".

An essential element in the plan is that the Government would be required to guarantee to keep health expenditure, from which the health vouchers would be funded, at least at current levels in real terms. Thus the value of the vouchers would be protected against general inflation. If the economy were buoyant it might be possible to increase health spending at a faster rate, accepting that it could account for a rising proportion of *total* public spending which was itself being reduced as a percentage of a growing national income.

On balance, I believe health expenditure should continue largely to be funded in the same manner as it is at present, with roughly 83% coming from the Treasury's Consolidated Fund and 13% from NHS contributions — although there may well be need for a change in the mechanism through which about 3% is now obtained from charges. Whether or not it would be advisable to retain the framework of the existing funding system is an issue which should be examined before the other changes are implemented. To keep it would preserve the element of equity which is the basis of our taxation arrangements and to which people, rightly, attach importance. The alternative would be to fund health expenditure through a separate and dedicated fund.

It would clearly be necessary for the Government, after the allocation of health vouchers, to retain central funding for a number of purposes. It would still have to accept responsibility for some services which would not be supplied by the authorised providers, either at all or to an adequate level. The extent of these services would, again, be something which needed detailed examination but the most important would be medical education, training and research.

There would also be a section of the community which it would be unreasonable to expect the authorised providers to cover. The precise definition of this group, to which I will refer as the "government insured" (no doubt it would be possible to find a better term), is another area which will need examination and, certainly, tough negotiating with the providers or insurers. Essentially they would be the chronic sick and the long-term mentally ill. The insurers would argue that the category should include more (e.g. all pensioners) and it would be in the national interest for the Government to agree to less (by no means all pensioners are bad medical risks — in the United States, for example, 45% of those over 65 do not use the health services at all in a given year).

The system would require an arrangement for medical boards to decide in particular, contested cases whether an individual should enter the government insured category. It would clearly be desirable to keep to the minimum the need for individuals to appear before medical boards to be classified but I believe that the arrangement would shake down fairly quickly so that in most cases the insurers and a National Health Authority, acting on behalf of the Government, could agree on the appropriate classification without the need of an appearance at a board. One way of keeping things simple would be to accept that all those over the age of, say, seventy would automatically fall within the government insured category — but the actuarial implications of setting any particular age limit would need careful examination. The treatment and care of this group would be without financial limit, subject to normal monitoring and proper medical authorisation under arrangements made by the National Health Authority.

A lot of work will be needed to put hard figures on these proposals but it would at least facilitate their further examination here to proceed on the basis of an estimate. My own calculations suggest that it would be reasonable to work on the assumption that the health voucher would have a value of at least £300 in 1987–88 terms. During that year NHS spending *per capita* was £373, of which spending on training education and research accounted for £18. For the reasons explained above, it is impossible to put a precise figure on the amount which the NHA would be likely to need for the government insured but the available data suggests that it could leave more than £300 per head for the rest of the population.

At first sight this is not a large sum when account is taken of the rates currently charged by companies in the medical insurance field and the relatively restricted nature of the cover they offer (for example, GP treatment is usually excluded). It is here, however, that the insurance principle will, I believe, come to the rescue. The new system will open up a huge market over which the costs will be spread; at present the great majority do not receive treatment costing anything approaching £300 each year.

This point is well illustrated by the figures for gross expenditure in England in 1987 on hospitals, community health and family practitioner services per head of population[2]:

Age	£	Population (mid-1984 in '000's)	Live & Stillbirths (mid-1984 in '000's)
Births	1,155		604
0–4	245	2,955	
5–15	140	6,808	
16–64	160	30,160	
65–74	495	4,048	
75+	1,075	2,986	
All ages	265	46,956	

There would be a need for wide consultation on the implementation of the voucher scheme as there are a number of other issues which would need to be resolved. For example, there would obviously be advantages for the administration of the scheme to issue a single flat-rate voucher to every individual in the insurable category. The insurers, on the other hand, could argue for a multiplicity of rates — depending on age, sex, medical history and, probably, area of residence (e.g. London weighting). With a flat rate system the insurers would compete for the best risks (the young and fit) and would be reluctant to accept voucher holders who were older or who had a worse-than-average medical history. It should certainly prove possible to find a satisfactory arrangement

— after all the DHSS already has experience in setting a variety of capitation fees for general practitioners. It might be enough to have two rates for the insurance voucher, that is to say — in 1987 terms — one below and one significantly above the £300 figure. The higher rate might be for those over 65 or with a poor medical history and the lower rate for the remainder. Actuaries and medical experts could make the necessary calculations without too much difficulty. Many categories, with the increased need for medical boards and the classification of individuals, would complicate the system to an unnecessary and intolerable extent.

I do not believe that a specific London weighting need prove to be either justified or necessary. An important element in the higher hospital costs that obtain in London is that which arises from the teaching and research activities of a number of London hospitals. Under these proposals such expenditure would be funded centrally (and probably more generously). Another major cause of higher hospital costs in London is a much greater propensity of general practitioners there to refer cases to hospitals than is the norm in other parts of the country. I believe that the proposals I set out below on the arrangements for primary care will relieve unnecessary pressure on London hospitals.

The realities of human nature and the experience of medical systems in many countries point to the need to create some mechanism which will involve the individual directly with the cost of his medical treatment. In some countries the patient pays a fixed percentage of the cost of his treatment, in others the first tranche of the costs, sometimes fixed on an annual basis. Some such mechanism would improve the effectiveness of these proposals and this is another issue which should be settled in negotiation with the authorised insurers or providers. Special arrangements could be made for those on low incomes on the lines of the exemption they are granted at present from the payment of prescription charges.

So much for the outline of the new funding arrangements. For the provision of health care, at the primary level, I would see the emergence of three different types of arrangement in the first instance — although I would expect others to evolve over the years.

The common and essential element is that, in return for the annual payment of the voucher, the new system would provide or assume financial responsibility for all necessary treatment, including hospitalisation and specialists. The major alternatives would be general practitioners operating broadly on present lines but supported by insurance cover; some form of health maintenance organisation or full medical insurance taken out by individuals. Which particular arrangement prospered would, in the end, depend on the judgement of the public exercising the freedom of choice it would enjoy in allocating its health vouchers.

At least in the first few years of the new scheme, I would favour positive steps by the NHA to promote the development of health maintenance organisations. This is likely to be necessary to combat the innate conservatism of most general practitioners. As we noted in Chapter Eight, the HMO concept has a long history, takes a number of forms and has not been without its critics and its problems. However, a series of studies indicate that, at their best, HMOs deliver good quality care which is sensitive and responsive to the needs of the individual. They have an incentive to promote preventive medicine and "wellness" programmes and avoid unnecessary hospitalisation (the Rand Corporation study, referred to on page 136, showed a reduction of 40% in in-patient treatment).

There is already a trend for GPs to work together in larger group practices and establish "health centres" with many more facilities than can be found in the traditional surgery. This provides a useful basis for the development of fully-fledged HMOs equipped with a wide range of testing and diagnostic facilities and the capability of carrying out minor surgery. Such facilities would do much to relieve the burden on expensive hospitals and patients of the need to travel to, wait in or be admitted to them — although care would be needed in the early years about minor surgery by a generation of general practitioners with no experience of it. Minor surgery which goes wrong can be major surgery; one safeguard here would be the financial incentive on the GP to avoid the risk of expensive treatment at a later stage in the case.

I believe that, in the longer term, the HMO concept offers the best prospect for developing high and steadily improving standards of health care. For the patient it would provide "managed care" and "wellness programmes" — approaches rarely found in the NHS — and it would enhance the contribution made by the general practitioner, enabling him to fulfil much more effectively the role of "gatekeeper" of the health service which has always been claimed for him. To use the jargon of the health economists, HMOs place "utilisation control" in the hands of the doctors rather than, as is largely the case in the NHS, of the administrators. Experience overseas shows that HMOs do not have waiting lists and that they are particularly good at caring for those who would fall within the "government insured" category I have defined above.

In his study, *Good Health: The Role of Health Maintenance Organisations*, Dr Eamonn Butler quotes an impressive quantity of research into the American experience with HMOs which demonstrates that, far from surrendering to any temptation to provide inadequate care to patients in order to increase their own returns, they actually provide care that is *better* on most measures than that available from other delivery systems. Butler also records "the persistent finding that the quality of care, as measured by a range of indicators, was better for people from poor backgrounds and those with apparent high need for care and treatment. In other words, not only do HMOs provide cheaper care, but they provide it more willingly to the poor. Not only do they provide better care, but they target it more accurately at those who are in need of it."[3]

The Government should therefore look for ways to persuade general practitioners to set up HMOs. One possibility would be one-off grants, on the lines of existing practice-improvement allowances, to promote the equipment of health centres on the lines discussed above. It might also make sense to offer tax concessions to newly-formed HMOs — although I am always reluctant to introduce new artificialities into the tax system. These are all possibilities which need to be examined.

Once the move to HMOs got under way it could be expected to gather a momentum of its own. It is likely to be helped by at least some of the companies already in the field of health insurance, just as in the United States the Blue Cross and Blue Shield plans have been active in the promotion of HMOs. I would also expect new enterprises to develop as public appreciation grew of the benefits which can be offered by HMOs.

Many general practitioners would be reluctant to join, however, and this could have advantages by offering the consumer a range of choice. Some GPs, having spent all their working lives in the special position of "independent contractor" created by the NHS, would be averse to becoming involved with the larger operation of the HMO and all that it entails. In any case, there would be serious practical difficulties for those working in the more remote country areas as experience in other countries suggests that the minimum size for an effective HMO is probably about 30,000 patients.

Doctors who elected to continue in traditional general practice would still operate under the system I propose. They would receive the value of the health vouchers from their patients, in return for which they would give the same guarantee as the HMO to provide or pay for the health care the patient would need. To protect themselves against cases which turned out to be very expensive they would be able to take out the sort of "stop loss" insurance which is well known in some countries. Such insurances might either be effected at Lloyds or, possibly, with the National Health Authority itself.

Some general practitioners would be apprehensive about the administrative and financial implications of the new system. I believe that, in practice, they would not turn out to be onerous. Many GPs already have "practice managers" working for them who could certainly handle the work which would be involved. I am also certain that management service agencies would be developed to offer administrative support to GPs who needed it.

The third major alternative method of arranging for primary medical care would be for the individual to use his health voucher to take out health insurance, probably on a fee-for-service basis. There is no doubt that the insurers, spurred on by competition, would develop a wide range of options from which the customer would be able to choose. It is likely that many would be variations of the arrangements for the Preferred Provider Organisations which have emerged in the United States as alternatives to the HMOs and which were discussed in Chapter 8. Private insurance would give the patient greater freedom to make his own decisions about his health care than would be possible under the other arrangements.

A fundamental element of the system I am proposing is that the individual, whilst retaining the guarantee of health care at least as good as that offered by the NHS, would have a range of choice and alternatives which is, at present, denied him. It is the conventional view in the medical profession that this is not an area where the ordinary citizen is able to make sensible choices — but I am sure that this patronising attitude is increasingly outdated. Greater competition produces more information — which, in turn, improves the individual's chance of making better choices. Patients would therefore have the right to change their provider or insurer but, for a number of reasons, there would need to be some restriction on the frequency with which they could do this. In some countries with systems similar to the one outlined here, they are allowed to do so every three months. I suggest that six months would be a reasonable minimum period. Providers would not, in normal circumstances, be able to refuse to accept any patient who applied to them. In any disputes in such cases, the NHA would act as the arbiter.

As already noted, a system on these lines carries a number of built-in safeguards which would ensure that a good quality of care was delivered. These safeguards would be reinforced by a general supervisory role exercised by the NHA, which would, for example, monitor such things as waiting times for hospital treatment.

A crucial requirement of the new system would be a capacity to stimulate the nation to spend a higher proportion of its increasing wealth on health care. This would be achieved by "topping-up" the health vouchers to buy benefits additional to those which would be provided against the health voucher. Under the standard arrangement, for example, all decisions on care would be taken by the HMO, with little or no patient freedom. To obtain greater freedom and options such as private hospital rooms, the choice of time for

treatment or the possibility of cosmetic surgery many people would
be prepared to top-up their health vouchers and hence generate the
additional funding that health care in Britain needs so badly.

I believe the marketing efforts of the insurers and the HMOs
would quickly generate growth in this sector. Employers, recognising that they benefit from a workforce which is kept fit and
treated well when ill, would have an incentive to top-up health
vouchers. It would also be a means of attracting and retaining staff,
particularly when the benefit was extended to the employee's
family. "Topping-up" would become an entirely normal and accepted part of an employment package, rather than the elitist
arrangement it tends to be at present. Trade unions could be
expected to add their own pressure — as would wives, who might
well urge, for example, spending rather less on the family holiday
in order to pay more for high-grade health cover. Whilst recognising the point I made earlier about the general undesirability of
further complicating the taxation system, tax benefits for top-up
payments, either by the individual or the employer, is another area
which deserves further examination as a means of stimulating more
spending on health.

Overseas experience — and the high priority which people
understandably give to their own and their families' health —
suggests that once the new system is introduced it would be
strongly supported. The insurance schemes in Belgium, for
example, offer five different levels of cover and benefits. Only 1%
are on the basic level, whereas 45% have chosen the most expensive.
Given the safeguards and controls suggested above, the more
money that is spent on health care, the higher will be the level of care
provided — and that would include the care of those who do not
top-up their health vouchers.

These proposals would create the opportunity to restore local
hospitals to the control of the local community, a long-held
ambition which has never yet been realised because of the funding
problems which are involved. I believe that under the new arrangements the hospitals could simply be handed over — lock, stock and
barrel — to the local community, however defined (and many of us

are sensitive about the horrors committed in the name of the "community" which was so much in vogue in the 1960s). It would be simple enough to establish them as economically viable but (probably but not necessarily) non-profit making entities on the pattern which exists in many other countries.

Careful consideration would, of course, be needed about the bodies which should take over what are, by any standards, major enterprises. The average general hospital has a capital value and a revenue account which both run into tens of millions of pounds.

My own suggestion is that each hospital should be placed in the hands of a board of trustees on which would sit representatives of the existing District Health Authority, the relevant local authorities (from County and District) and of the medical, nursing and related professions. The three groups should have roughly equal representation and the Chairman in the first instance would be appointed by the Government.

Once appointed the trustees would be invested with total *personal* responsibility for the hospital and its conduct. My suggestion would be that the National Health Authority draw up a model trust deed (to deal with such matters as the replacement of trustees) which individual hospitals might wish to adopt but I believe this is a matter on which each locality may well wish to work out its own arrangements. My only caveat would be that hospital boards should be insulated from the political wrangling that has caused such problems in local government in recent years.

When established, the hospitals would be run on a commercial basis, competing with hospitals already in the private sector to provide the services required by the HMOs or authorised insurers. Pay levels, recruitment, investment and all the other decisions which are now made or strongly influenced by the DHSS or the Regional Health Authority would be in the hands of the trustees.

With a network of autonomous hospitals there would be no need for the 192 District and 14 Regional Health Authorities, whose abolition would lead to significant savings in manpower and resources. As I noted earlier, in 1985-86 these authorities in England alone had administration costs of £374 million. This would be more money for the health vouchers. It would also, regrettably, be likely to add to the chorus of criticism which will, inevitably, greet these proposals. The RHAs and DHAs will not go down without a howl of protest.

I propose that there should be a National Health Authority, independent of government, to oversee this structure. It is not an essential element of the plan — the role could be fulfilled by the DHSS or the existing Health Service Supervisory Board — but it would have the great merit of largely removing the health issue from the political dog-fight. No doubt there would always be pressure on the Government of the day to increase the health budget and the value of the health voucher but for the rest the lines of responsibility and control would be very much clearer than they are now.

The idea of some sort of independent "Health Corporation", perhaps on the lines of the BBC, has been under discussion since at least the 1940s but has always foundered on the difficulty inherent in the conflict between independence and the need for account-ability to the public through Parliament for a publicly financed service. I believe the proposed arrangements largely overcome that problem. The Minister of Health would be responsible to Parlia-ment for centralised health spending and the level of the health voucher, whilst his relationship to the National Health Authority would be analogous to that of the Home Secretary and the BBC.

The general functions of the NHA have, I believe, already emerged in the foregoing. It would monitor the system to ensure that patients are given proper treatment and would arbitrate in the matter of complaints against the providers or the insurers. It would have a range of sanctions at its disposal, from fines to the with-drawal of a licence to operate. It would vet and approve HMOs and insurance schemes and their arrangements for such items as co-insurance or "excess" charges for treatment. It would arrange the medical boards which would be needed to decide on the "govern-ment insured". It would assist in the launch of NHS hospitals into their new and autonomous role and in the creation of HMOs. The NHA should also monitor the provision of what are known at present as regional or supra-regional services and, should it prove necessary, stimulate their provision. I think that in practice the new system will generate its own demand for such specialised and high-grade facilities — and will be much better able to meet that demand than is the NHS.

The creation of the NHA would be an opportunity to bring the voices of the medical, nursing and related professions into the national consideration of health provision in a much more constructive manner than we have seen in recent years, due to the fact that the structure of the NHS has forced them into an antagonistic relationship. The authority should not be dominated by the professionals — but they have a vital role to play.

One final thought. From the beginning, the NHS was criticised for its failure to create a *unified* service, providing little or nothing in the way of after-care, rehabilitation, domiciliary care for the elderly or chronic sick, nursing homes etc. Over the years, some of these responsibilities have been taken up by the social services departments of local authorities and others — such as nursing home payments for those with little capital — by the social security budget of the DHSS. In some areas, such as after-care, we provide virtually nothing and compare very unfavourably with many other countries. In some instances three budgets — NHS, local authority and DHSS — overlap expensively. In others there is a gap and no provision of services. There is a constant battle between central government, the local health authority and local government about who should pay for what, which has been at its most bitter in the struggles over the concept of "care in the community". This whole area is a long-standing mess which has become even worse as tensions between central and local government over funding issues generally have increased in recent years.

In very round terms, using 1987 figures, all these activities account for some £4,000 million of public money through the various budgets, spent for the benefit of about 10 million pensioners and chronic sick. It would be possible to issue this section of the population with a second voucher at the rate of about £400 each — or even to spread the money more thinly over all the age groups —

and set up an arrangement with licensed providers to organise the services which are needed. This structure could also be subject to monitoring by the National Health Authority and would be likely to provide a better and more co-ordinated service to the elderly and the chronic sick than they have at present. This is one more area which deserves careful examination — with a readiness to contemplate much more fundamental changes than are, I believe, being considered by Sir Roy Griffiths in the review of community care he is completing at the time of writing.

A New Chapter

We have come to the end of this book but I hope we are at the beginning of a new chapter in the creation of an adequate system of health care in this country. The debate has begun, as the nation has finally come to question whether Bevan's creation, supported on all sides for forty years, was the right prescription.

The danger now is that, in the traditional British manner, we shall fudge and tinker rather than reform. It is a time for boldness and courage. The health and welfare of the British people demand nothing less.

At the head of the penultimate chapter of his book, *The Development of the London Hospital System 1832-1982*, Geoffrey Rivett offered a quotation from Machiavelli. I am sure it is one that is still more appropriate to these proposals:

> ... there is nothing more difficult to arrange, more doubtful of success, and more dangerous to carry through than initiating changes ... The innovator makes enemies of all those who prospered under the old order, and only lukewarm support is forthcoming from those who would prosper under the new. Their support is lukewarm partly from fear of their adversaries ... and partly because men are generally incredulous, never really trusting to new things unless they have tested them by experience.

References

CHAPTER ONE

1. J. Enoch Powell, *A New Look at Medicine and Politics*, Pitman Medical Publishing Co. Ltd., London, 1966, p.16.
2. *Ibid.*, p.67.

CHAPTER TWO

1. Michael Foot, *Aneurin Bevan*, Vol 2, Davis-Poynter, London, 1973.
2. Quoted in Harry Eckstein, *The English Health Service*, Harvard University Press, London, 1959, p.161.
3. *A National Health Service*, HMSO Cmd. 6502, 1944, p.6.
4. John E. Pater, *The Making of the National Health Service*, King Edward's Hospital Fund for London, 1981, p.7.
5. Geoffrey Rivett, *The Development of the London Hospital System 1823–1982*. King Edward's Hospital Fund for London, 1986.
6. Rudolf Klein, *The Politics of the National Health Service*, Longman, London, 1983, p.9.
7. Public Records Office, MH 80/24. Minutes of "The first of a series of office conferences on the development of the Health Services", dated 7 February 1938; Minutes by the Chief Medical Officer, dated 21 September, 1939.
8. Sir William Beveridge, *Report on Social Insurance and Allied Services*, HMSO, 1942, para 437.
9. *Ibid.*, para 267.
10. *Ibid.*, para 437.
11. Eckstein, *op. cit.*, p.139.
12. Cmd. 6502, *op. cit.*, p.9.
13. *Ibid.*, p.8.

14. *British Medical Journal*, 1944, Vol I, p.295.
15. Michael Foot, *op. cit.*, p.17.
16. Klein, *op. cit.*, p.17.

CHAPTER THREE

1. Public Records Office, CAB 129/3, Memorandum by the Minister of Health: "The Future of the Hospital Services", 12 October, 1945.
2. Public Records Office, CAB 129/3, Memorandum by the Minister of Health: "The Hospital Services", 16 October, 1945.
3. Hansard, House of Commons, 5th Series, Vol 422, 30 April 1946, Col. 66.
4. Commons Hansard, 15 February 1946.
5. Eckstein, *op. cit.* p. 163.
6. CAB 129/3, *op. cit.*
7. Public Records Office, MH 77/73, Letter dated 18 July, 1946.
8. Commons Hansard, 30 April, 1946. Col. 43.
9. Commons Hansard, 30 July, 1958. Col. 1383.

CHAPTER FOUR

1. Public Records Office, CAB 129/38, National Health Service: Control of Expenditure, Memorandum by the Minister of Health, 10 March, 1950.
2. Powell, *op. cit.*, p.27.
3. Richard Crossman, *Paying for the Social Services*, Fabian Society, London, 1969.
4. Public Records Office, CAB 129/131, The National Health Service: Memorandum by the Minister of Health, 13 December, 1948.
5. Public Records Office, CAB 134/518, Cabinet Committee on the National Health Service: Enquiry into the Financial Working of the Service — Report by Sir Cyril Jones.
6. Quoted by Michael Foot, *op. cit.*, p.337.
7. Klein, *op. cit.*, p.51.
8. Department of Health and Social Security, NHS Twentieth Anniversary Conference, Report, HMSO, London, 1968.
9. House of Commons, Social Services Committee, 4th Report 1985 — 86(HC 387): "Public Expenditure on the Social Services".

CHAPTER FIVE

1. National Council for Social Services and King Edward's Hospital Fund, *Voluntary Service and the State*, 1952, p.125.
2. Klein, *op. cit.*, p.84.
3. *The Times*, 18 December, 1987.

CHAPTER SIX

1. DHSS Memorandum: NHS Scrutiny Programme 1983 — Residential Accommodation.
2. Alain C. Enthoven, *Reflections on the Management of the National Health Service*, London, 1985.

CHAPTER SEVEN

1. *Universities Work for Health*, Universities Information Unit, London, 1987.
2. *Health: The Politician's Dilemma*, OHE, London, 1986, p.7.
3. Robert J. Maxwell, *Health Care UK: An Economic, Social and Policy Audit*, London, 1984, p.127.
4. Henry J. Aaron and William B. Schwarz, *The Painful Prescription: Rationing Hospital Care*, Brookings Institute, Washington, 1984, pp. 91-94.
5. Reported in *The Times*, 4 January, 1988. Source: IMF.
6. Office of Health Economics, Compendium of Health Statistics, 6th Edition, 1987.

CHAPTER EIGHT

1. David G. Green, *Challenge to the NHS*, IEA, London, 1986.
2. Harold S. Luft, *Health Maintenance Organisations: Dimensions of Performance*, New York, 1981.
3. *Measuring Health Care 1960-1983*, OECD, Paris, 1985.

CHAPTER TEN

1. *British Medical Journal*, 10 October, 1987.
2. Commons Hansard, 25 February, 1987, Cols. 331-2W, OPCS Population and Vital Statistics, 1984.
3. Dr. Eamonn Butler, *Good Health: The Role of Health Maintenance Organisations,* Adam Smith Institute, London, 1986.

Index

Addenbrooke Hospital,
  Cambridge, 90
Addison, Dr Christopher, 20,
  21, 24
Administration Costs of NHS,
  86
Aids, 14
Alcohol, additional duty, 131
Ambulatory Surgical Centres, 120
Area Health Authorities, 62, 72,
  75
Attlee, Clement, 32, 44, 56
Australia, 122, 132

Belgium, 94, 100, 126, 132, 154
Bevan, Aneurin, 17, 30, 32,
  Chapter 3, 46, 55-58, 65, 79,
  105, 111, 125, 141, 145
Beveridge, Sir William and his
  Report, 28-30
Blue Cross, 115, 119, 152
Blue Shield, 115, 119, 152
British Medical Association, 20, 21,
  38-40, 47, 48, 52, 63, 64, 82,
  142, 145
British Medical Journal, 23, 31,
  98, 103, 145

Brittan, Leon, 76, 77
Burgess, Mark, 6, 13

Canada, 102, 124
"Care in the Community", 69
Castle, Barbara, 73
Cave, Lord, and his Committee,
  24
Central Medical Board, 31, 39
Central Policy Review Staff (The
  "Think Tank"), 76, 77
Chamberlain, Neville, 25
Citrine, Sir Walter, 40
"Cogwheel" reports, 70
Community Health Councils, 72
Competitive Tendering, 87-89,
  128
Conservative Government, 61, 63,
  72, 75, 83, 87, 90, 96, 128
Co-payments, 116, ,124, 126
Coronary heart disease, UK and
  US comparisons, 121
"Cost improvements", 91
Cranbrook, Earl of, and his
  Committee, 69
Cripps, Sir Stafford, 32, 57
Crossman, Richard, 50, 71, 91

Daily Mirror, 7, 10, 83
Daily Telegraph, 11
Dalton, Hugh, 32, 34
Dawson, Lord (of Penn), and his
    Report, 21-24
Diagnosis Related Groups
    (DRG's), 94, 114-115, 132
Dialysis Services, 140
District General Hospitals, 75
District Health Authorities, 70,
    82, 92, 135, 155
District Management Teams, 72,
    78
Doctors, numbers of, 99

Elliott, Walter, 26
Emergency Medical Service, 26,
    28
"Emergicentres" (in the U.S.),
    120
Ennals, Lord, 18
Enthoven, Alain C., 92
Epstein, Joseph, 3
Executive Councils (for GPs), 68

Family Practitioner Committees,
    72, 76
"First Green Paper", 71, 141
Foot, Michael, 17, 32
Fowler, Norman, 77
France, 94, 97, 99, 102, 103, 126,
    132, 134
Frimley Park Hospital, 53-54

Gaitskell, Hugh, 46, 57
"Gatekeeper" role of GPs, 67,
    151
Germany, 97, 99, 100, 102, 103,
    123, 134
Gillie, Dr Annis, and his
    Committee, 69

Goldsmith, Dr Michael, 136
Graham Little, Sir Ernest, 30
Greenwood, Arthur, 34
Griffiths, Sir Roy, 62, 78-79, 105,
    158
"Group Model" HMOs, 117
Guillebaud Committee, 58-59, 68,
    69

Guys Hospital, 6

Haldane, Lord, and his
    Committee, 20
Harrow Health Centre, 136
Havard, Dr John, 48
Hayhoe, Barney, 63
Healey, Dennis, 104
Health Maintenance
    Organisations (HMOs),
    116-119, 135, 136, 150-153, 154,
    155, 156
Health Service Management
    Board, 78
Health Service Supervisory
    Board, 78, 156
Health spending, 98, 101-105
Holland, Stuart, 18
Horton, Sir John, 30
Hospital beds, numbers of, 99,
    100
Hospital Management
    Committees, 66
"Hotel Charges", in NHS
    hospitals, 91, 128
Howe, Sir Geoffrey, 76, 142
Hughes, John, 140

Independent Practice Associations
    (IPAs), 117-118
Institute of Health Service
    Management, 63, 64

"Internal Market" in NHS, 92, 128

International Monetary Fund, 61, 102, 104

Jones, Sir Cyril, 56
Jones, Dr Ivor, 142-149
Joseph, Sir Keith, 72, 91

Kinnock, Neil, 5-6, 10, 141
Korner Committee, 92

Labour Cabinet, 34, 40, 46, 65, 79, 108
Labour Party, 5, 32, 35, 37, 39, 40, 44, 57, 58, 61, 72, 73, 111, 125, 139
Land sales, of NHS property, 90
Law, Richard, 36-37
Liberal Party, 77
Lloyd George, 19, 20, 38, 111, 125, 139, 145
Lotteries, 133-134

MacNalty, Sir Arthur, 27-28, 34
"Managed Care", 116, 120, 151
Maude, Sir John, 27, 68
Maxwell, Robert, 7, 83, 100
Maynard, Professor Alan, 93-94
Medicaid, 113-114
Medicare, 113-114
Mental Health Act 1959, 69
Merrison, Sir Alec, 73-74
Messer, Sir Frederick, 35
Ministry of Health Bill 1918, 20
Moore, John, 9, 10
Moorfield Eye Hospital, 85
Morrison, Herbert, 32, 34, 37, 65, 79, 108, 125, 139, 145

National Health Authority proposal, 147, 150, 152, 155-156

National Health Insurance Bill 1911, 19
National Health Service Bill 1946, 18, 36, 42
National Health Service Contributions, 60, 74
National Health Service Reorganisation Act 1973, 72
National Insurance Contributions, 130, 146
Netherlands, 99, 103, 123
"Network Model" HMO's, 117, 119
Newton, Tony, 11
New Zealand, 111, 122
Nursing staff levels, 97, 98

Paige, Victor, 79
Patients First, 75
Peacock Committee, 133-134
Pharmaceutical Prices, 59
"Planning, Programming and Budgetting" (PPB), 60
Plowden Report 1961, 60
Poor Law, 19
Poor Law Hospitals, 25
Porritt, Sir A., and his Committee, 69
Powell, Enoch, 13, 15, 41, 50, 51, 76
Preferred Provider Organisations (PPO's), 119, 153
Private beds, in NHS hospitals, 72
Private Health Insurance, 95, 113, 128, 154
Private Patients Plan, 136
"Programme, Analysis and Review" (PAR), 60
Public Accounts Committee, 62
Public Expenditure Survey Committee (PESC), 60

Quality Adjusted Life Years
    (QALY's), 93

Reconstruction, Ministry of, 24
Redcliffe-Maud, Lord, 71
Regional Health Authorities, 72,
    74, 82, 135, 140, 155
Regional Health Councils, 72
Regional Hospital Boards, 66
Resource Allocation Working
    Party (RAWP), 59
Robinson, Kenneth, 71, 141
Royal Colleges of Medicine, 11,
    39, 73, 82
Royal College of Nursing, 63,
    64, 82, 96, 98
Royal Commissions: on the
    Health Service, 73; on Local
    Government, 71; on the Poor
    Laws, 19

St Thomas's Hospital, 5, 18
Salmon Committee, 70
"Second Green Paper", 71, 72
Seebohm Committee, 71
Silkin, John, 72

Smith, Cyril, 77
Spain, 100, 134
"Staff Model" HMO's, 116-117
Summerskill, Dr Edith, 29-30, 59
Sweden, 102, 103, 124-125
Switzerland, 99, 103

Thatcher, Margaret, 1, 5, 6, 9, 10,
    12, 15, 76, 77, 85, 91, 107
"Ticket Moderateur", French
    system, 126, 132
Tobacco, additional duty, 131

United States, 86, 97, 102, 103,
    109, 112-122, 134
Utley, T. E., 50

Walker-Smith, Derek, 41
"Wellness" Programmes, 121,
    127, 151
Welsh Health Authority, 140
White Paper on the NHS, 1944,
    18, 28-31, 58, 141
Willink, Henry, 29, 31, 32, 34, 37

Young, Sir George, 75